GILLES MONIF, MD

# Bellevue Diary

Lights within the Shadows

iUniverse, Inc.
Bloomington

iUniverse books may be ordered through booksellers or by contacting:

iUniverse
1663 Liberty Drive
Bloomington, IN 47403
www.iuniverse.com
1-800-Authors (1-800-288-4677)

Because of the dynamic nature of the Internet, any web addresses or links contained in this book may have changed since publication and may no longer be valid. The views expressed in this work are solely those of the author and do not necessarily reflect the views of the publisher, and the publisher hereby disclaims any responsibility for them.

ISBN: 978-1-4620-0845-2 (sc)
ISBN: 978-1-4502-9025-8 (ebook)

Library of Congress Control Number: 2011904972

Printed in the United States of America

iUniverse rev. date: 07/19/2011

# Contents

## Part III  A3: First Medical Division

## Part IV  B4: First Medical Division

*Preface*

## Fred

The first day of anatomy was a personal challenge that could not be avoided. The bodies had to be carried up from cold storage in the basement to the Anatomy Dissection Room. Death had yet to touch my life. Though family members involved in the French resistance had died in World War II, I had never before been physically exposed to death. When volunteers were asked for, I took the first step forward. After carrying thirteen bodies up three fights of stairs, their collective weight blunted my initial fear.

Having volunteered, I got to choose the cadaver that I and three other classmates would dissect. I chose a thin white male, probably in his sixties. Having established a truly physical relationship, I named him Fred. In the many hours we spent together, Fred shared glimpses into his life with me. The skin of his hands told of hand work. His lungs, two sacks filled with coal dust, spoke of where he had been. The near absence of fat and his body's donation by the City of Boston to the medical school bore witness to the probable poverty of his last days.

In teaching me about the human body, Fred opened my consciousness to, not death, but the steps before it.

*Bellevue Diary* chronicles more than just a tribute to a great institution. The events related are nonfiction. They occurred primarily between 1961 and 1962, the year of my medical internship. The names of most individuals have been changed; for several individuals, not to recognize them would be wrong.

The lights within the shadows provided the insights that allowed me to write, "You meet many persons who desperately cling to lives that have long lost their substance. Physical existence is the last possession they have. And then there are those who come to death with 'their cups filled.'" Before I too enter into the shadows, I want to share experiences that enriched my life.

*"The people that walk in darkness have seen a great light: They that dwelt in the land of the shadow of death, upon them hath the light shined."*
Isaiah 9:2

# Part I
*Bellevue Hospital*

## Bellevue Hospital

In 1736, Bellevue Hospital, the oldest public hospital in the United States, was founded. At the time, George Washington may have been four or five years old.

Following a fire that occurred sometime around the turn of the century, between 1906 and 1939 Bellevue was rebuilt in bits and pieces. She now shows her age: a conglomerate of brick buildings stretching along First Avenue from Twenty-Fifth Street to Thirtieth Street. The one architectural element that gives her an illusion of grandeur is the Administrative Building, which faces First Avenue. Its strong, vertical, inlaid concrete columns take one's gaze upward to a pseudo-Athenian temple facade that towers two stories above the adjacent roofs.

What makes Bellevue great is that she is the hospital from which "no one is turned away." She is an open-ended funnel into which New York dumps its poor, elderly, and dying. If an individual presents at another hospital for admission and it is apparent that he or she will demand a disproportionate amount of care, the admitting physician has only to write "No beds" and the patient is Bellevue-bound.

Competition for internships at Bellevue Hospital is intense. Its 2,500 patient beds are the medical equivalent of what was once the great library at Alexandria. Within each bed, a potential lesson waits—a lesson in which knowledge is exchanged for a dose of healing. Educationally, big-city hospitals are the Harvards of the medical world, and, as at Harvard, learning can come at a steep price.

The Medical and Chest Services are divided between three medical schools: Columbia University (since 1888), Cornell University (since 1888) and New York University (since 1898). Each institution has imparted to its house staff a unique profile. The Cornell interns and residents are dubbed the "All-American boys." By and large, they tend to be clean-cut and have the distinction of having been elected by their respective school faculties to the national honorary society, Alpha Omega Alpha (AOA). The New York University interns and residents emphasize academic brilliance over decorum and appearance. The Columbia interns and residents are called "the aristocrats of Bellevue." The latter image is largely fashioned by the predominance of Columbia graduates among its house staff. They are New York's response to the proper Bostonians.

My reasons for wanting to be part of the Columbia Medical Service had to do with something else. The Columbia Medical Service at Bellevue had produced more academicians than even the Thorndike Service at Boston City Hospital. In the 1950s, a Nobel Prize in Medicine had been awarded to its director and his collaborators for pioneering research in the area of pulmonary physiology. What I did not know when making my selections for the National Internship Matching Program was that his retirement was imminent.

The Chief of Service's replacement seemed a strange choice: an uptown physician whose patients had, more likely than not, frequented Harkness Pavilion at Presbyterian Hospital. At Bellevue, the patients, more often than not, called the Bowery home.

Despite having graduated in the top ten of my class and having very strong letters of recommendation, the absence of my election to the national honorary medical society should have raised a red flag. My election to Alpha Omega Alpha had been blackballed by two professors.

## The Room

The house staff rooms are located on the fifth and sixth floors of the Administration Building. Five cartons of medical books and two suitcases of clothes quickly teach me that, at Bellevue, the elevators are more symbolic than functional.

Tired from carrying the last load of books up five sets of stairs, I quickly turn the key, push the metal door open, and begin carrying the items stacked outside the door into the room.

The light filters through the dingy, double-hung window that opens onto a ventilation court. The room is ten by twelve feet, if that. Immediately to my right is a built-in closet that can be opened only if the door is closed, giving the remaining room a nine-by-ten-foot configuration. A simple metal desk and chair, a metal bed, a sink, a two-by-three-foot mirror, a sixty-watt bulb on the ceiling, and a telephone compete for the remaining space.

Before unpacking, I start cleaning away the debris left by its former occupant: detached front covers of medical journals and loose sheets of notes written in a tight, careful scrawl. The dust on the desk and windowsill outlines where other books had been.

The single central desk drawer jams for a second time. With difficulty, I extract a small wad of paper that had been wedged in the drawer. In a scrawl I already know is written:

*When you come into contact with a man,*
*no matter who, do not attempt an objective*
*appreciation of him according to his worth*
*and dignity. Do not consider his bad will,*
*his narrow understanding or perverse ideas,*
*as the former may easily lead you to hate*
*him or the latter to despise him; but fix your*
*attention on his suffering, his need, his*
*anxieties, his pain. Then, you will ...*

The rest had been torn off.

## Doubts

It's dark. I lie fully clothed, motionless on the bed. The outlines of the room's furnishings are barely visible in the reflected light coming through the window.

A little over three weeks ago, I was a medical student, with little true responsibility for patient care. The ultimate decision had always been someone else's. Tomorrow morning, that will all change. I will put on white pants, a white shirt, and a white jacket. To patients, the resultant vision is an illusion suggesting some sort of immaculate conception. They rarely see the very prominent feet of clay.

The lack of sleep last night loses its foundation. At the meeting for the new house officers that day, the piece of paper with my name on it states that my medical internship is to start in Siberia, otherwise known as the Chest Service. My adrenal rush fades.

# Part II

*The Chest Service*

## The Chest Service

The Chest Service is the relatively recent name given to what had previously been known as the tuberculosis wards for the city of New York; now, in 1961, tobacco's gifts to the human race have changed the character of its occupancy list. Looking forward to repetitive encounters with tuberculosis, lung cancer, and chronic bronchitis and emphysema is not my idea of happiness.

What makes starting out on the Chest Service a really bad deal is that an internship in the Columbia Medical Division is part of a pyramid system in which there is no guarantee of a tomorrow. Twelve interns are selected annually for the Columbia Medical Service. At year's end, only six will be offered a first-year residency position. When I rotate off the Chest Service and into the Columbia Medical Service, my performance will be judged primarily against former Columbia students, who will have already had three months of relevant experience on the medical wards.

## FUO

Twenty charts are mine to review. By tomorrow morning, an on-service note summarizing the key medical problems needs to be in place in each chart. At chart nineteen, repetition's monotony is interrupted.

Stephano Fassio is a twenty-nine-year-old Sicilian cook, who for the past two and a half months has been running fevers of unknown origin (FUO) between 102 and 104 degrees. His body has literally melted from 198 pounds to an emaciated-looking 145 pounds. His condition has already made him the centerpiece of medical grand rounds uptown, both at New York and Presbyterian Hospitals. Despite extensive scrutiny, his diagnosis remains unchanged: fever of unknown etiology.

The chart makes fascinating reading, until I reach the previous resident's off-service note, which states that Stephano Fassio is to be transferred to the Columbia Medical Service in preparation for presentation to a visiting professor at the next medical grand rounds.

Stephano Fassio is the jewel in the package of charts assigned to me. I raise a masssive storm of discontent with the Chest Service's chief resident. He brokers a compromise. Stephano Fassio's transfer will be delayed until just before grand rounds, provided that everything possible is done to find out what is slowly killing him.

My on-service note covers five single-spaced pages. In exchange, Stephano Fassio stays.

All his medical information is based on the initial patient interview. The problem is that Stephano Fassio does not speak English. His story had been obtained using an Italian interpreter. Stephano Fassio is Sicilian. Italian and Sicilian do not necessarily mesh.

That night I walk down to a bar in Little Italy. The address was given to me by one of Bellevue's security guards with connections.

"Where can I find a Sicilian who …" receives an initial blank stare from the bartender.

"Get the fucking …" has just enough time to escape his lips when a deep baritone voice asks, "What do you want a Sicilian for?"

The body language of the two guys at the bar tells me that I am treading in deep water.

I now face a man who is dressed in an elegant three-piece black suit with thin blue stripes—a marked contrast to my jeans and sweater. Surprisingly, the man appears to have been listening carefully. His penetrating gaze is answered, but probably not for the same reason.

I tell him the story of Stephano Fassio rather quickly. I hand the man a card with my name, the chief resident's name, the attending physician's name, the hospital's address, the telephone numbers, and, lastly, Stephano Fassio's name.

The man asks if I want a drink. I respond that all I want is an interpreter. Looking at the now-interested observers who have edged closer, all I probably really want is out.

On the walk back to Bellevue, I console myself. At least I tried. Back to plan number two.

Plan number two is trying every conceivable unused diagnostic procedure. In one of my medical books, I had read that patients with retroperitoneal lymphomas, when given a substantial amount of alcohol, often experience abdominal pain. The next day, I am dealing with a completely smashed Stephano Fassio, singing at the top of his lungs while trying to dance with a nurse's aide, who is trying, without much success, to get him back to bed. The book never stated how much alcohol was required. There is going to be hell to pay for this fiasco.

Before I can act, the ward nurse interrupts me. "I've been looking for you. There is someone here to see you."

I follow her out into the corridor. Seated on a straight-backed green metal chair is a slender girl, probably fifteen to sixteen years old, in a high-collared pink and white cotton dress. The man from the bar stands next to her.

With hesitation, she slowly gets up. She takes two steps; her hand extends forward as if in slow motion. In it is the card. "I'm Sicilian." Her voice is barely audible.

Unconscious, stroked out, or senile, speaking Yiddish, Chinese, Spanish, Hungarian, or God knows what, Bellevue's unique clientele rolls through its doors, challenging you to figure out on your own what is real and not real. A famous physician named William Osler once said, "Let me take the history and let anyone else do the physical examination, and I will give you the diagnosis in 80 percent of the cases." The language barrier disappeared as Stephano Fassio told her the story of his disease; and then she told it to me.

Three hours later, a probable diagnosis is in place. Diagnostic tests are ordered. When finished, the Chest Service's chief resident's phone rings.

Three days to get past "go." I am excited. The next day, I can't wait to get out of clinic and check to see if any of the tests are back. When I get to the ward, Stephano Fassio's bed is empty. The freshly pressed sheets announce that he is

11

not returning. The chief resident of Medical Services for the Columbia Division had used his leverage to have Stephano transferred. With a VIP visiting professor, the Division is taking no chances on a subpar presentation by a new, untried intern.

If the Chest Service's chief resident is pissed, he hides his emotions well. "If it's any consolation, they were impressed with your workup," he says in a consoling tone. "It got us two possible concessions."

There is no missing the use of the word *us*.

"Firstly, you may or may not be asked to comment before the visiting professor dissects the case, and …" And then comes a long pause. "Oh, yes. If by any chance we establish the diagnosis, Fassio comes back to the Chest Service." The smile at the corner of his lips says it all.

As I start to get up, the chief resident of the Chest Service hands me a familiar piece of paper. "By the way, the last page of Stephano's chart appears to have been misplaced. Give this to the ward secretary and have her forward it to First Division."

Given the internal inefficiencies inherent in the system, that piece of paper will not be reunited with its chart anytime in the near future.

Two days of data preparation are just that. The night before an ego battle is to be waged for possession of Stephano Fassio, we slowly consume two cups of the best Turkish coffee that $1.35 can buy.

First Division's monthly medical grand rounds are a big deal. The auditorium is filled to standing-room capacity.

The First Division's chief resident gives a very comprehensive, detailed presentation, followed by a lengthy summary of all the previous medical discussions.

Finally, the prayed-for misstep occurs. "Does the Chest Service have anything to add?"

As rehearsed, the Chest Service chief resident motions for Stephano Fassio to be wheeled in. Once in place, Stephano Fassio's previously untold story of muscle and joint pain is presented. His subdued cry of discomfort when his triceps and calf muscle groups are compressed speaks to the veracity of diagnosis. Then come photomicrographs from the skin-muscle-nerve biopsy, slides of the electromyelogram, and, finally, the reading of an unofficial consultation from one of the NYU's rheumatologists.

Without discussion, fever of unknown origin becomes fever of known origin. Stephano Fassio has polymyocytis, an inflammatory disease of the muscles and joints.

For what is probably just a few seconds, nothing. Finally, the squeak-squeak of the wooden wheelchair breaks the auditorium's silence as Stephano Fassio is pushed home to the Chest Service.

## Double Jeopardy

The previously hot political frying pan got hotter.

The new director of the Columbia Medical Division has made a reputation in the field of rheumatology with the use of corticosteroids, drugs that reduce inflammation. When the order that steroids are to be used is transmitted down the chain of command, another brief firestorm breaks out.

Stephano's chart contains two instances in which his temperature had precipitously dropped to normal and stayed there for approximately four to five hours. In each case, he had been given a single aspirin. Large doses of antipyretics had produced only a partial response. When the final push of authority is applied, Stephano Fassio goes to First Division, but not until he has been without fever following twenty-eight hours on a regimen of one adult aspirin every four hours.

He does great on low-dose aspirin. Two months later, I am asked to write, as the coauthor, a draft of *Treatment of Polymyocytis with Low-Dose Aspirin,* which is to be my first academic publication.

Only after everything is really over does reality creep into my consciousness. Victories leave behind the vanquished, who do not necessarily forget and perhaps don't forgive.

## The Gift

My junior-year medical school roommate gave me the gift of assassination with two-by-two slides.

After five generations, John was the first of his family to have escaped the Welsh coal mines. Despite his talent and brains, he was nearly relegated to spending his entire life in the mines. When he won a scholarship to a university, he almost did not take it. His family was not in a good position to lose the money he was making in the mines.

At the university, John became a star swimmer. In time, he made the 1950 British Olympic team as an alternate. There, he met the Yale University swimming coach, who brought him to the United States.

Not having completed his degree in England, he needed to get a degree if he was to become a head swimming coach. At Springfield College, he found that his interest had gone beyond sports. As a junior, he applied to Harvard. They turned him down, but Boston University did not.

If space is available, the best students from Boston University are occasionally allowed to do their senior elective in medicine on Harvard's Thorndike Service. John and I were so chosen.

My supervising intern is a great guy with a good sense of humor. He likes to play mind games. John is not as lucky. His intern is a pompous ass who still has not recovered from having been passed over by Massachusetts General Hospital. When he is not being one, he is kissing one.

Just before the rotation ends, God gives John a gift. His intern had a patient with a severe Group A beta-hemolytic streptococcal wound infection. Despite many days of penicillin therapy, cultures of the wound continued to demonstrate the persistence of the organism. The intern became excited. He was convinced that he had something big and arranged to make a special case presentation to the chief of the Thorndike Medical Division.

Two days before the big show, John asks me to join him in the service's laboratory. "Look under the microscope and tell me what you see."

"Clusters of small gram-positive cocci consistent with streptococci," I reply.

"Now look at this slide and tell me what you see," he says, removing the slide and replacing it with another.

I move the microscope objectives to a lower power to be better able to scan the slide. Three seconds latter, I am back to high power. "I'll be damned! You've got lots of streptococci, but staphylococci are also present."

Removing the slide from the microscope, John says, "The staphylococci are protecting the streptococci by breaking down the penicillin before it destroys the streptococcal cell wall. Everybody has been taking cultures from the center of the wound. Slide two comes from just beyond the edema border. If you can get the projector from histology, I'll get photomicrographs developed."

John's intern elects to make the entire presentation and, in so doing, walks the plank. Traditionally, the medical student presents the case. This fact is not wasted on Dr. Kass, who asks, "What does the medical student have to add?"

Before John can answer, his intern quickly intervenes. "He is a BU student!"

John, using his best Welsh accent, takes command. "May I have my first slide."

He then precedes to document in great detail every error of thought and action completed and omitted.

We may have been the first BU students to ever be given a going-away party. Apparently, we were not the only ones whom said intern had pissed off.

## Good Offense, Bad Defense

Stephano Fassio was a great start for me on the Chest Service, but within a month, the Cornell intern and I are wondering if we are the two dumbest interns in the hospital.

Every day for the past three days, questions have been asked on rounds that expose minor gaps in our charts: an incomplete white blood cell count, an unchecked box. While not serious deficiencies per se, the frequency with which they surface appears to document preparation deficiencies.

The Chest Service is a specialty service shared by Cornell University, New York University, and Columbia University. Brad, the Cornell intern, was AOA out of Maryland. George was third in his class at Albert Einstein.

On day four, George brings up a very minor point about the occupational history of one of my patients. I realize that there is no way anything related to that had been previously presented. *The son of a bitch has been reading my patient charts!*

War is war! George has been very good at offense, but how good is his defense?

Day five, every third patient of his is taken apart on attending physician rounds.

Day six, his chart deficiencies on every second patient of his are exposed in detail.

Day seven brings about capitulation and the beginning of a friendship born out of gamesmanship and defensive skills that suck.

Despite its limited menu of teaching material, the Chest Service has become fun, largely due to the quality of its attending staff and the relatively light workload compared to that of my medical counterparts. Being on call only every third night allows for time to prepare for when I will go on to the medical wards, as well as other pleasures. The catalyst for the latter is the general cafeteria, which, by unspoken agreement, is the meat market for student nurses, nurses, and male house staff.

## Tobacco's Addictive Grip

Fighting tobacco's addictive grip is too often a study in masochism. We rarely get big victories. Last week, I had a chronic bronchitic patient admitted in $CO_2$ narcosis. It takes three days in the iron lung to give him back the ability to breathe without assistance. As soon as he can ambulate, off he goes to the bathroom. While sitting on the toilet, he smokes until he again loses contact with his surroundings.

The week before that, while on night shift, I notice a bright, little red light irregularly flickering in the darkness.

The problem isn't that the patient is smoking. The problem is he is smoking in a damn oxygen tent. That the patient and I are both alive is a testimony to the excellence of Bellevue's oxygen tents.

## The Social Order

Learning the social structure at Bellevue comes quickly. Yesterday, an attending physician and I went rummaging in the sub-basement under the K and L buildings for usable parts for Bird Respirators. The Bird Respirator is a medical respirator for acute or chronic cardiopulmonary care that was invented during World War II to enable pilots to fly planes at high altitude.

Our arms filled with assorted pieces of equipment, we got into the freight elevator. Four maintenance workers and a nurse's aide had apparently elected to take the trip down to the sub-basement. The elevator stopped at the basement floor. There stood another maintenance worker with four enormous trash barrels.

Opening the elevator door, the corpulent operator sitting on her elevated stool turned to us and said, "Doctors, you have to get off. We have garbage to load."

They are the permanent staff. We are but transients in their world.

## Left Breast Coat Pocket

Every Wednesday, we have a radiology conference. The most challenging chest X-rays of the previous week are presented as unknowns for a given resident to diagnose. This particular day, the intern from the Cornell Service is not getting it. Finally,

Dr. McLain gives up, asking, "What's wrong with this X-ray? Brad, where is the cancer on this X-ray?"

Brad has failed to notice a subtle change in the take-off of the left main stem bronchus. The pressure to answer correctly is evident. The vein in the middle of Brad's forehead is bulging. Suddenly, looking straight at Dr. McLain and not the X-ray, he bursts out laughing. *"Right there,"* he says, pointing to a pack of cigarettes in Dr. McLain's left breast coat pocket.

He doesn't know how right he is.

## The Dining Room

The dining room is open for three meals a day, plus a fourth meal between 11:00 p.m. and 1:00 a.m. For those on the medical and surgical services, making two out of four meals gives better odds than three out of four.

Though the house staff knows little about the kitchen staff, the kitchen staff knows much more about us than just our names. This knowledge will occasionally be made evident by selected individuals getting an additional piece of steak on those rare Sundays when others are being chased out the kitchen's door with, "Can't you read, doctor? No seconds!"

Six months later, this is all made clear. Mrs. Grady's mother is admitted to A-3 with specific instructions.

Mrs. Grady runs the dining room and, apparently sometimes, the medical administrator. The hand-written note accompanying the admission slip spells out in no uncertain language exactly who are to be her doctors.

## A Journey Not Kept

Yesterday, a comrade on the Chest Service died a little.

Salvatore Cusumano smoked his first cigarette when he was ten and never stopped. He smoked until he could no longer work; until a block became a mile; until he had to stop several times when yelling orders to his wife or daughters; until the day his lungs were so damaged that they could no longer rid themselves of the metabolic waste, carbon dioxide. When the concentrations of this gas reached critical levels and his lungs failed to oxygenate his blood adequately, Salvatore Cusumano's heart failed and his sensorium succumbed to what we call $CO_2$ narcosis.

Salvatore Cusumano was unconscious and cyanotic when Carter entered the picture. The peach-fuzzy appearance of youth belies Carter's true character. When no special duty nurse was available, he gave up several of his free nights to make sure the old man was still there in the morning.

When Salvatore Cusumano regains consciousness, his first cry is for a cigarette. It takes a long time and a lot of patience for Salvatore Cusumano to mend. The degrees of improvement correlate directly with his verbosity. By the time he is sitting in a wheel chair, he is yelling, "Go away! Don't torture me anymore. Let me die in peace!"

Carter just smiles and goes about doing what he thinks best for his patient. The shouts and protests are of short duration. In the ensuing weeks, a real fondness appears to develop between the two of them.

The day Cusumano is to be discharged, Carter is tied up with an emergency. Salvatore Cusumano will not leave until they have said good-bye. He had his wife bake a large Italian bread, studded with glazed fruits. While his family waits downstairs, he sits in a chair with the enormous bread in his arms, waiting.

When Carter appears, Cusumano gets to his feet, but suddenly his face becomes crimson, then purple. His neck veins bulge. He slumps to the floor.

As I start downstairs to tell the family that Salvatore Cusumano will never be going home, I look over my shoulder to the end of the corridor. Carter is leaning against the wall, his face buried in his arm.

## Peking Duck

The recent frequency with which potatoes and noodles appear on the menu means that another budgetary shortfall has occurred. With the end of the chest rotation coming up, three of us will be pooling our money. The much anticipated meal is Peking duck. Not any Peking duck—great Peking duck. The question is where.

Finding great Chinese food means finding the right cook. In Chinatown, a new restaurant starts by hiring a master chef and offering his creations at relatively nominal prices. Once the reputation of the restaurant is established, the chef moves on and the prices move up.

Before our money is spent, we will make a number of visits to Chinatown. We will seek a Chinese restaurant that on a week night is filled with Chinese patrons. Once a number of non-Chinese patrons is readily visible, the master chef has left, and great Chinese food becomes good Chinese food.

The Chest Service has been fun and maybe a little too easy.

# Part III

*A3: First Medical Division*

## Doubts

Sleep does not come easily. Music helps, but tonight I need something more. Renewed doubts demand my attention. Tomorrow I will finally become an intern on First Division's Medical Service.

In the past, reading nonmedical books has helped. Piling two pillows, one on top of the other, on the bed, I grab a book of famous essays from those stacked upright on the desk.

Page fifteen of Voltaire's *Essays* is the wrong choice!

*Doctors are individuals who prescribe*
*drugs, of which they know little.*
*For diseases of which they know less,*
*In human beings of which they know*
*nothing.*

A poster that contains the Promise of the Circle is the sole decoration in the room. Tonight, reading it out loud helps.

*Walk with me through the darkness and I'll*
*lead you to the light.*
*Walk through the storms of adolescence*
*and the summers of manhood shall be yours.*
*Walk through the gardens of triumph and*
*failure and I will lead you to the Northern*
*Lights of wisdom.*

## A-3

My first rotation is on First Division's only female ward, A-3. A-3 could have doubled for a ward of an early Victorian hospital. It's a large, open room with fifteen-foot ceilings; the furthermost windows look out onto the East River. Rows of beds line each wall, and two additional rows of beds, head to head, occupy its center. A series of eight-foot-tall windows breaks the southern wall. The nurse's desk is at the front of the ward. From there, she can survey all the beds.

Every morning, fail none, A-3, A-4, and B-4 medical patient rounds begin at 7:00 a.m. A large metal cart containing the patients' medical charts is pushed down the aisles separating the rows of beds. The cart stops at the foot of each patient's bed on its right.

The attending physician and the patient's intern move to the head of the bed. A brief conversation and/or examination ensues, after which the entire group, composed of the attending physician, two second-year residents, four interns, the ward nurse, and medical students and nursing students, reunites at the foot of the bed. There, his or her disease, treatment, progress, and, not infrequently, prognosis are discussed. At a private hospital, these discussions would be held outside of a patient's room. But this is Bellevue. Six feet buffer the group's conversations from the patient. Unwanted and sometimes irrelevant information can be had for the listening.

Between the beds are small metal stands; the drawers are a patient's sole claim to privacy. If a patient has any fears or apprehensions, they are destined to be heightened by what is around them. Neither mascara nor rouge can hide the anguish and despair or the ultimate consequence of life. The only time portable curtains appear is either for a procedure or for preparing the bed for its next occupant.

The patients could probably live with the covers pulled over their heads, but that would do little for the occasional smells coming from neighboring beds.

## Night Sounds

The first night on the ward is different from anything that I experienced on the Chest Service.

If day is reality on A-3, night is not. Most of its occupants are drawn primarily from the geriatric populations of New York. They are sundowners, ranging from pre-senile to the frankly Loony-Tunes. In a familiar environment, they can function reasonably well. Take them out of that environment, put them in a hospital setting, take away the modality of sight that darkness imposes, and they do not have the mental reserves to compensate. They become disoriented, frightened, and sometimes violent: children of regression, lost in the night.

To the sundowners, add a group of stroked-out patients. A few of these have fixated on a single sentence or group of words, which is all they can say. And they say it all day—and sometimes all night.

The night sounds include the hum of a respirator, the hacking cough of Kathleen McGill, the "aie, aie, aie" of

Carmen Rodriguez, the "O Lordy, Lordy, save me" of stroked-out Bessie MacGray, responding to the broken Yiddish of Rebecca Horowitz.

The night sounds get to someone. Out of the darkened ward comes, "If they don't shut up, I'm going to kill them."

The sequence of sounds becomes so funny that I am about to start laughing, when, from somewhere in the darkness, a shrill voice cries out, "My God! She's dead."

## The Touch

The first night, death does not finish its work early. B-4's on-call intern and resident are tied up in the emergency ward. They need someone to pronounce Morton Goldstein dead.

Morton Goldstein is a thin, white-haired male, somewhere in his late seventies. His body temperature is dropping. There is no respiration; no heart beat. His blood pressure is unobtainable. His pale blue eyes are still open, but if there is a clue to his last moments, it has long since disappeared. I fold the slender arms across his breast.

After filling out the forms that officially certify him as dead, I leave the ward.

In the next hour, I become uncomfortable. Is he really dead?

Morton Goldstein is still in the long corridor leading from the B-4 ward: wrapped like a mummy in white paper that is bound by white tape, awaiting his delivery to the morgue. For reasons that defy knowledge, I need to tear away the paper and feel the cold certainty of death's touch.

## Emergency Room Baptism

The emergency room baptism is unforgettable.

The call box in the hall pages me to the emergency room. I run down three flights of stairs, through a corridor, and across the parking lot between the A and B buildings and the emergency ward.

One of the emergency room nurses intercepts me in the hall and tries to explain, but she almost doesn't have to. The high-pitched screams and shouting coming over the metal partition that screen the emergency room from the corridor tell the story, but not with quite the same adjectives.

Magdalena Mariotti, the matriarch of a large Italian family, has been admitted in marked respiratory distress. Her reaction to her inability to catch her breath is hysteria. Like a contagious disease, hysteria has quickly spread to the four other members of her family present. When the nurse and an orderly try to relieve Mrs. Mariotti of her numerous layers of clothes, they are pummeled from all sides.

After reviewing the admission notes, I make my entrance on what is by then the fifth chorus of, "Oh, mamma mia, I can't breathe!" to which the chorus responds, "Oh, mamma mia! Mama can't breathe! La poveretta. La poveretta!'

The visual picture matches the sound track. My introduction to the group requires more than a little shouting.

At full voice, I announce, "I have come to help your mother. She is now in my care." Almost in the same breath follow the words, "You need to go to the waiting room. *Now*!"

After glancing at la mamma for their cue, over a thousand pounds of human flesh depart. That leaves me with 275 pounds in the rotund form of Magdalena Mariotti.

As she starts on the sixth chorus of, "Oh, mamma mia, I can't …" I cut her short. "I can sing louder than you."

She bursts out laughing. Then we go from comic opera to something more serious.

## No Problem, Big Problem

The time required for an internal medicine workup varies depending on a number of factors: the severity of the disease, the number of diagnostic procedures required, and above all, the little blank boxes in the chart. At night, the intern does the urine analysis and blood work. If anemia is documented, protocol demands that a sternal bone marrow biopsy be done and a preliminary reading of said be recorded. Unfortunately for the interns, a low red blood cell value is epidemic in populations subjected to poverty, disease, or blood-letting for money. If an electrocardiogram is needed, three guesses as to who does it and records a preliminary interpretation in the chart. If an X-ray is indicated and the patient comes in at night, you are the porter. In short, you can count on an average of two to three hours of concentrated effort per patient.

A second-year resident from one of the four medical divisions usually screens potential admissions to the medical wards. Once accepted, the patient is admitted to the appropriate service next on the rotation; however, if that patient had previously been on a given medical service, that takes precedence over the rotation. Not uncommonly, the admitting resident of a given service, seeing that the impending admission is a readmit to his service, will strategically misplace the old chart and have the individual admitted to the next service in the rotation.

The absolutely worst possible scenario for an intern is when the admitting resident is from a support service, like radiology or psychiatry. Specialization tends to contract their medical knowledge to a point where anything that they do not understand gets the benefit of a bed.

Tuesday goes well: five patients. Only one patient comes in at night. The presentations during morning rounds are precise. The charts are immaculate. Not a single little blank box has escaped nurturing.

Thursday, I have one admission during the day and two that night. Finishing the last workup at 3:45 a.m., and with preliminary rounds starting at 6:00 a.m., I figure that it's not worth getting so little sleep. For two hours, I read.

Friday morning's attending rounds go well. So far, so good. One admission at 4:00 p.m ... no problem. No problem, either, when the second comes in at 5:55 p.m. and the third at 6:45 p.m. Still not a big problem when number four rolls in at 7:37. Between 9:00 p.m. and 5:00 a.m. numbers five through nine are wheeled onto the ward.

"No problem" evolves into a mind-bending nightmare. The little boxes on which my performance will be evaluated kick my butt physically and mentally, to a point where I almost don't care.

The night before, I forgot to finish packing. Charlie, one of my friends from the Columbia Surgical Service, and I are to be ushers at a mutual friend's wedding. The pre-wedding dinner is to be in Washington DC Saturday evening.

At 11:25 a.m. on Saturday, my answer to his "Where the hell have you been?" is to throw Charlie a box of latex gloves and a tube of KY jelly. In the next twenty minutes, someone will push a finger into the anuses of seven of Bellevue's finest so that all the little blank boxes are feed.

In the months to come, I become good at catching a fifteen-minute nap while leaning against a wall. Given the choice between sleep and sex, the word with the most letters wins more than its fair share.

## Checks and Balances

Each division's services from the three medical schools eat at their respective tables. Cross-fraternization is unusual. The services literally war against each other in a game of determining who is best. If and when a mistake is made, one or more of the house staff from a competing service will make certain that you know that they know. It is Bellevue's system of unspoken checks and balances at work.

Five Columbia Division house staff members are sitting at a dining room table when Ira comes up. It quickly becomes an uncomfortable moment. Ira has blown a diagnosis. An elderly bronchitic patient had been admitted with respiratory distress. Not understanding the disease process with which he was confronted, he had treated her for pulmonary edema. The therapy for one condition can be lethal for the other.

As he sits down, Will, from Second Division Medicine, walks over and caustically inquires, "Seen any bronchitics lately?"

Ira just looks down at his plate. Two of the Columbia interns abruptly terminate their dinners and leave. He has disgraced the service.

I stay, but not out of desire. Sometime, somewhere, I will walk in those shoes.

If you ever meet an internist or surgeon who says that he or she has never killed or contributed to the demise of a patient, he or she is either a dermatologist with a limited scope of practice or an individual in acute denial of reality.

We are all 007s—only licensed by society rather than Her Majesty's Secret Service.

## Mine or Theirs

Black on white. The roach looks up from the sheet. The cracking and peeling of the paint on the ceiling breaks the silence. Sweat is pouring off me as I strip down and lie on the narrow metal-frame bed. There may be a breath of air somewhere outside, but here, within this inner quadrangle, the heat is stifling.

The hell with it! I get up and grope for the towel with which I have already wiped off a day's perspiration. With it wrapped around my waist, I walk down to the john. The cold tiles are a welcome change. This john was built in 1937. The showers probably broke down in 1938; there is little evidence that they have ever been repaired.

On the sixth floor, there is no such thing as a cold shower. It is either a scalding hot shower or none. Someone has scratched into one on the metal doors that lend privacy the words *illegitamae non-carburandim*: Latin for *Don't let the bastards grind you down*. Nobody has ever seen fit to paint over it.

After a cursory transit through Hades's Little Geyser, I'm back in my room, responding to my name being paged. I slip on my white pants, shirt, and jacket. I still get a tremendous kick out of them. As I lace up the white shoes, I notice two small bloodstains. With that sick humor fatigue breeds, I wonder, *Mine or theirs?*

Right now I'm numb with fatigue. This week I've been on duty 109 hours; but the figure that really counts is that this shift has only four more.

## VIP Rounds

Attendance by the Columbia off-service interns at the First Division's medical grand rounds and VIP medical rounds is mandatory. This particular morning, "the grand old man" has come down from Presbyterian to do morning rounds. Though well into his seventies, his mind has the quality of vintage wine. But his tongue has the capability for vivisection of those manifesting deficiencies of knowledge.

Any grubby mode of dress is gone. Our white coats and pants are immaculate. Everybody stands straight. To be caught leaning against a bed is an invitation for verbal castigation. Well, almost everybody is straight. Toward the end of the first hour, Bill begins a series of tell-tale gyrations, shifting from one leg to another.

Chronic urinary retention and chronic constipation accompany an internship at a big-city hospital. To survive, you learn the location of every john and facsimile thereof. Today, Bill has apparently omitted performing a prophylactic piss after morning coffee.

With the changes of bed sides, his predicament guides him to the periphery of the group. When everyone's attention is fixed on the case being presented, he carefully lowers himself to the floor and disappears under the adjacent bed.

A few minutes later, the discussion ends. The entire entourage of thirty or more medical students, nursing students, interns, residents, nurses, and attending physicians now moves in the same direction that I had seen Bill scampering on his hands and knees. They encircle the last bed on that row.

Under the pretext of picking up a pen, I confirm that Bill's trip to the bathroom will have to wait a while longer.

## Schwarzewolke

Reality is challenging enough without what Levi calls "Schwarzewolke" (a better term: Kleine-Schwarze plague).

Last week, I had had three young ladies in their late teens to mid-twenties convinced that they had brain tumors.

Why? The previous night, they had individually shared a religious experience on the idiot box. They had watched

Benji Schwarzewolke, otherwise known as Ben Casey, MD, brilliantly (Madison Avenue's term for self-evident) diagnose a brain tumor in a nineteen-year-old girl. With a clinic full of really sick patients, what should be funny doesn't register.

## Not My Job

Big-city hospitals tend to be cesspools of neglect in many ways. For some, working there is a convenient niche in which to pass time until payday. Accumulated over twenty or more years during which they have been underpaid and treated like second-class citizens, some have come to a poor compromise between their potential and their level of commitment. Even those individuals whose compassion or comprehension motivates them to a greater sense of personal responsibility often find it difficult to sustain that commitment in the face of the ridicule and the inertia of peers. "Only a sucker works!"

Attempts to reform are of limited value. They know that they will be here long after I'm gone.

Today a cardiac arrest occurred on the B-4 ward. A cardiac arrest becomes a total consumption of all trained personnel, in which the time and intensity of your involvement may translate into the survival or death of that patient. Before racing from A-3 to help, I ask the porter cleaning the floor if he'd remove the bedpan from under an elderly patient when she gets through.

Almost an hour later, I walk on the ward, tired, frustrated by defeat, only to find her in tears. The iron rims have taken their toll.

Carrying the goddamn bedpan, I walk over to the porter, who is courting one of the nurse's aides at the other end of the ward. "I thought I asked you to remove this!"

"Man, that's not my job. I'm only paid to clean the floors."

Seconds later, the contents of that bedpan unceremoniously empty themselves onto the floor.

## Fecal Impaction

The likelihood of getting the residency seems more and more remote. It's primarily my fault. Imprinting is not necessarily limited to ducks. My father admired Mahatma Gandhi a great deal. For Gandhi, "There is no God higher than truth."

In retrospect, I come to realize that we may not always see the world or ourselves directly. What we tend to see is ourselves as mirrored by others. In the mirror, right is might. In the real world, might is right.

Having been raised with strong parental mirrors, I have the dangerous tendency to push against the grain of perceived truth a little more than is prudent and not respond to fear. In medical school, it cost me election to AOA.

My frequent reassignment to A-3 indicates that I don't exactly fit First Division Medical Service's prototype. That knowledge frees me from concern about the future.

Most of the interns, particularly the male interns, prefer working with male patients. Female patients require pelvic examinations. That, in turn, requires that a female attendant be present, which introduces a big scheduling problem and adds a lot of extra time to the workup. But the biggest thing that redirects enthusiasm away from A-3 is the words *fecal impaction*.

Over age sixty, the intestines don't always listen to their owners. When patients are over seventy and receive certain drugs that tend to depress intestinal motility, a more liberal use of prune juice or milk of magnesia is often necessary. Over eighty, communication between intestines and performance sometimes requires a *deus ex machina* in the form of an index and middle finger.

The first time that I had to deal with that problem left a lasting impression.

Having finished attending physician's rounds, I had just sat down to finish my daily patient progress reports when the ward nurse interrupted me. "Dr. Smithwick and his resident are both in clinic today. Can you take care of Mrs. Copnicki? She's impacted!"

Distracted for the moment by the little blank boxes, I reply, "Put the curtains around her and I'll be there in a moment." The word "please" seemingly has gone on a temporary vacation.

She looks at me for a moment longer than usual. "This is your first fecal impaction, isn't it?"

In response to my head nod, she says, "I'll get you a nurse's aide to help." She hesitates. "Never mind. I'll take care of it myself. You had best do this in the treatment room and not on the ward."

To me, fecal impaction means a plug. At Bellevue, fecal impaction means having to dislodge a massive consolidation of hardened feces, which, at times, has you thinking "Hoover Dam."

Her last recorded bowel movement occurred five days ago.

"I suggest you give her morphine." I bow in compliance to a higher power. The morphine will make her constipated, but without it what is about to happen may not be humane.

An ointment with a local anesthetic is applied to the anal opening. I wait for it to take hold. Digital examination reveals a massively dilated rectum filled with rock-hard feces. The first attempt to dislodge a small portion elicits a scream that could be heard in San Francisco. But something comes.

The next few visits to the black hole bring forth unique four-letter words of endearment. I keep telling myself, this very vocal elderly lady is somebody's mother.

A half hour later, the bedpan is almost full. Then it happens. Liquid feces gush forth. The treatment table, my pants, socks, and shoes are re-colored brown.

The paging system, telling me that I have a new patient waiting for me just around the corner on the ward, almost drowns out her words. "Thank you, doctor. I feel wonderful!"

## Goya versus El Greco

Roger has just returned from the uptown ivory tower (Presbyterian Hospital).

"Well, how was it?" I say, sliding into the chair next to his, my tray loaded with the surprise of the day.

"The food is as bad as I remembered; but it's great to be back," he says, his mouth half full.

"The difference is like the two Saint Peters, one by El Greco, a tall elegant figure with the hands of a musician, and the other by Goya, a small pudgy figure with the hands of a peasant. The patients don't smell nor have lice! They are intelligent and articulate. But when you get through trying to look behind the facades, you don't have the feeling of being necessarily closer. Maybe I am just too used to raw guts to tolerate a calculated layer of veneer."

I jokingly reply, "Why don't you just say Bellevue is a place for those who prefer their Goyas to their El Grecos, irrespective of personal cost?"

At the time, I intended it to be a smart-ass remark. Once said, it had the ring of truth.

## Everybody Knows

Normally, a good deal of chatter accompanies the breakfast meal. Not today. A house staff member slips into a seat. Someone asks, "Do you know?"

Everybody knows.

At the top of the administration building, inside the Athenian-like temple, is a large room. Originally intended to be a house staff entertainment center, it stands largely abandoned. Two old ping-pong tables are there, without nets, balls, or paddles. Once a year, it hosts the house staff's Christmas party. The one thing that gives the room life or purpose is the soda-dispensing machine. When you are tired of tap water or cafeteria coffee, for ten cents you can buy a can of soda.

Last night, one of the surgical residents went there, apparently to do just that. Someone killed him: four stab wounds. He was in his surgical scrubs, which made it likely that the only money he had on him was just enough for the machine.

## Biggest Show in Town

The ambulance never actually stops. A surgical resident from the Cornell Service and I jump into the modified delivery wagon, with its seven-foot ceiling, that masquerades as an ambulance.

Saul has been driving Bellevue vehicles since the 1930s. He has seen far too much to get excited about anything. "Before you kids tear my ambulance apart, whatever you are going to look for, we don't have! So relax and enjoy the ride."

To, "Where are we going?" comes back a one-word answer: "Idlewild."

"What happened: a plane?"

"Spare me. A couple of idiot savants!"

For a while, we get little more out of Saul. He is too busy employing his talents on any vehicle that has the audacity to be on the same road and going in the same direction. He is right about one thing: with the equipment in this ambulance, we aren't going to be very effective.

The frequent stops (even though still in second gear), the grinding of gears coupled with liberal use of the king's

English (as interpreted through the Old Testament) give ample testimony to the fact that a major traffic jam is occurring.

Because of the heavy fog and the need to get the ambulances through, the police have blocked access to the Van Wick Expressway to all other traffic. Once on the expressway, you can't see more than twenty yards ahead. Saul is somewhat disenchanted when this is brought to his attention.

"Don't bug me. Go back and play dead or something."

I do, but after Saul sideswipes a lamp pole, I drive while Saul plays patient.

A police escort picks us up at the main entrance and directs the ambulance to the crash site. The smell of burnt flesh, plastic, and metal hangs in the air. There is nothing to do. There are no survivors.

I walk beyond the glare of the spotlights and look toward the wire fence at the perimeter of the field. Despite the fog, in the afterglow of spotlights, I can see what has to be thousands of people pressing against a half mile of chain-linked fence for a closer look. My stomach tightens. It must have shown. Saul puts his hand on my shoulder. "Kid, death is the biggest show in town."

## Coming Home

The telephone call makes no sense. "Your patient is in a private ambulance at the receiving station. Dead!"

The admitting resident meets me at the loading dock. "You lucked out! No big workup to do."

"I don't get it," I reply.

"Go speak to her son. He's in my office."

Saying that, he hands me the admission sheet. On it is her name, Sandra White, and corresponding address: South Hampton, Long Island.

Still in the ambulance, Sandra White lies motionless. Her body temperature tells me that she has been dead for at least two hours.

Steven White is somewhere in his late forties, well dressed, well groomed. There is no mistaking the strain and sadness on his face, but no tears.

"I'm terribly sorry about your loss, Mr. White."

His face is now visible only in profile. Looking at the wall to his left, he replies, "My mother had terminal cancer. Her medical reports are on that desk," pointing behind him and to his right.

His head never moves.

"Why Bellevue? Why have you driven 150 miles in her last moments?"

He replies, "That's the way she wanted it!"

Now he turns, and the tears come. His jaw trembles.

"Her maiden name is Jacobson. She was born on the Lower East Side."

He hands me a piece of paper. It is a birth certificate for one Sandra Jacobson, dated February 7, 1895. Place of birth: Bellevue Hospital.

## Oy, Oy, My Heart

At 2:30 in the morning, I have the dubious honor of meeting the geriatric gem of the Columbia Service at Bellevue. At five feet, with white hair and pale blue eyes clouded by mature diabetic cataracts, Mimmie Schwartz sits in her wheelchair, clutching the right side of her chest, crying out the words, "Oy, oy, my heart, my heart!"

A mammoth chart, weighing some twenty pounds, is on her lap: a depository attesting to her fifty-one previous admissions. Strategically placed atheromatous plaques in her brain have removed any hope of effective communication, so I delve into her chart.

With this admission comes a departure from her usual script. In between, "Oy, oy, my heart, my heart" is now sandwiched, "My stomach, my stomach."

Somewhere on page 473 of Mimmie's massive chart, I discover that someone has prescribed nitroglycerine tablets (just in case a real need ever arose for them). Mimmie may be a sundowner, but she knows a good thing when it comes along. If one pill is good, just think what five or ten might do: cause stomach cramps!

Having solved one problem, I soon have another. I cannot regulate her blood sugars. Everything I try meets with failure.

Sometimes at night, I go unto the unlit ward. Watching the patients in the dark can bring clarity to my thoughts. Last night, I arrived just in time to witness Mimmie skirt over her hospital bed rails and take off running, shouting all the while those immortal words, "Oy, my heart, my heart," with the night aide, Willie Mae Browning, all 240 pounds of her, attempting a semblance of pursuit.

Mimmie disappears into the ward kitchen.

I had previously explored the possibility that she might be getting food from an outside source, but I discarded the thought. No one visited her, and no food is ever left out in the kitchen at night.

When Mimmie's reappearance isn't forthcoming, I go into the kitchen to find out why.

Had it not been for the muffled noises, I might not have found her. Lost from sight, Mimmie Schwartz sits inside a large, tipped-over kitchen trash can, wolfing down the discards and garbage left from the day before.

## Bells Unrung

Intermixed with the banging on the metal door is "Get the hell out of bed!"

Waking from a deep sleep, my transition to sitting upright is less than graceful. The good thing is that I fell asleep with my clothes on. As I reach for the door handle, I glance at the small electric clock on the desk. It reads 2:17 a.m.

The now-open door reveals a committee of two, Charlie and his girlfriend Jody, an ER nurse. Sleep-induced confusion delays my protest.

"It's Bill." Jody doesn't need to continue. We all knew it would ultimately happen. "Marvin is downstairs with him in Charlie's room."

Bill looks like shit. His hair is greasy. His shirt is in the sink, soaking. The smell of vomit permeates the room. Two to three days' growth of beard speaks for itself.

Bill must have been the catch of his graduating medical class: good-looking, with curly blond hair, deep blue eyes, and a father whose practice was exclusively Harkness Pavilion. His wife, Sharon, matched his blond hair and blue eyes. To say that she is visual candy would not do her justice; that is where all superlatives abruptly end.

Bill's marital give-and-take is badly out of whack. Sharon has made little allowances for what an internship's physical, mental, and emotional demands entail. What she doesn't attempt to understand is that medicine is Bill's mistress. Out of necessity, he can cheat on his wife, but God help him if he cheats on his mistress. There had to have been many a night that Bill was lucky just to have been able to make the drive up the Eastside Parkway without falling asleep. Sharon's nightly demands have stripped him of his manhood.

Bill's most immediate needs are lots of coffee, a shower, a good night's sleep, and a sympathy lay.

## A Circus Team

For the second time in a week, a mistake had occurred. This time insulin, a drug that lowers the blood sugar, had been administered to the wrong patient. Mistakes will happen, but when the mistakes were uncovered, the response had been denial.

The incidents involved a group of student nurses who have acted like a three-ring circus. Any sense of humor was lost with their first few bad acts.

There is no restraint in what is said. Only toward the end of the diatribe do I become aware of how uncompromising the language has become.

In the ensuing month, things seem to change. There is no more talking to each other on rounds. Their conduct and even posture mirrors that of Mrs. Solbiki, their nursing instructor. Now, they know their patient's medical histories and also, sometimes, that something extra that tells you they really know their patients.

At the termination of their seven-week nursing rotation, an end-of-rotation party is traditionally held. Amid the cakes and paper cup are two posters, one addressed to the staff and the second with my name on it.

The second poster reads as follows:

We started A-3 the very first week,
As "circus performers" young and meek,
We worked and we worked to fill the bill.
But it seems our attempts were strictly nil.
Something was lacking, we know not what,
But shy and unsure we asked not a soul,
For advice or help to enhance our role.
While we continued to fumble, things

looking quite gray,

Until taken aside on that momentous day,

And instructed to crawl from within our cave,

To begin the new road which we'd have to pave,

Of being inquisitive, curious, intent,

After the lecture we knew what was meant.

So as a team, we planned strategy one,

Our fight for approval had just begun,

The days passed, the weeks slid by,

We continued to work, continued to try,

Till now we find ourselves at the end.

It's up to *us* which way we bend.

But we have no fear the way that will be,

We'll just remember our motto learned from thee,

Ours is not to do or die, ours is but to

Question *Why*."

Bellevue is an incubator for more than just MDs!

## Hubris

I have less than a week left on A-3 when Lucy Garcia is admitted.

Twenty-two years old, about five feet five inches tall, long jet-black hair, and big oval brown eyes, she makes a beautiful canvas, blemished only by her swollen ankles. The curved elegance of well-turned ankles is absent. In their place are pipe-like enlargements that fuse into her lower leg. She has been admitted from the clinic because of edema of the legs.

She presents an exciting diagnostic challenge. The principal differential diagnosis for bilateral peripheral edema is right-sided heart failure versus a kidney problem called nephrotic syndrome, in which an individual loses so much body protein in the urine that the integrity of the blood compartment can no longer be maintained.

There is no mistaking the fact that she has very significant pitting edema. The application of a finger to the skin overlying the bone leaves behind a deep depression. Her history and the physical examination quickly rule out heart disease. When the examination of the urine fails to demonstrate the presence of protein, the mental fun begins.

A faster than anticipated heart rate is consistent with a contracted intravascular compartment. The increased whiteness to the underside of her eye lids speaks of a chronic illness. Now the history of two to three bowel movements a day takes on added significance. If I am right, she is losing protein through her bowels. The disease entity that has a potential surface commitment of adequate capacity to cause such a massive loss of protein is called regional enteritis.

The next day, the diagnosis, without a list of other possibilities, is presented on attending rounds. The attending and I had already played cat-and-mouse too often. Instead of challenging the diagnosis, he says in a resigned voice, "I assume you already have the small bowel X-rays to prove it."

Two dollars to the night radiology technician had worked. The small bowel series confirms massive involvement of the ileum and sigmoid colon, diagnostic of regional enteritis.

The Second Division Gastrointestinal Service is on her case like a dog on a bone. They put a body protein called albumin with a radio-labeled tag into her bloodstream. Large amounts of the tag are identified in her feces.

Regional enteritis is one of those diseases we do not understand the hows or whys of. It is an impressive collection of letters behind which we hide our collective ignorance.

Lucy is given the wonder drug of the 1960s, corticosteroids, and I leave the ward for B-4.

Five weeks later, I get a call from A-3's senior administrative resident. "Do you remember Lucy Garcia?"

A little hesitant, I ask, "Why?"

"She died! She had regional enteritis, all right, but it was due to the type of tuberculosis you get from drinking unpasteurized milk. There was no PPD in the chart! I thought you would want to know!"

Guilt inundates me. My instinct for self-preservation surfaces. I want to scream out, "What about the Second Division GI Service who took over management of her case? They had her four weeks. Why didn't they do it?" But it doesn't work for me. My ability to make a given diagnosis stick became a barrier to a more complete analysis.

The steroids were the firing squad. The responsibility for her being there is mine.

The word *hubris* is a Greek word that means overbearing pride or presumption. A spirit born of prior successes cultivated by ego cost Lucy her life.

I had killed my first patient.

## Sugar-Coated Bagel

The decision to try to salvage her is not one that can be defended by logic. When I tell our head nurse that I want one of the student nurses to work with Bertha Cohen, the arching of her eyebrows tells me what she thinks of the idea.

Bertha Cohen is a vintage, sugar-coated bagel. In the vernacular, a *sugar-coated bagel* is an elderly, stroked-out diabetic from the Lower East Side. Her stroke has not only paralyzed her entire left side but has terminated her ability to speak.

The probable futility of what can be achieved with such a patient causes a certain amount of caustic humor to creep into the initial examination. There's just one thing wrong. Despite her inability to move her left side and her seventy-two years, her eyes turn on at the appropriate times during what is a very one-sided conversation.

January has been hell! During the time while Bertha was being conditioned for the day when she will hopefully be able to take her first step, ward bed capacity went from the legal limit of thirty-two to thirty-seven and then expanded to the point that patients were being housed in the hallway and boarded out on other wards. The geriatric population explosion forces me to try to find a foster home for Bertha.

Her student nurse braids her hair and ties bright yellow ribbons at the ends. For the second time, Bertha is sent to the rehabilitation ward. For the second time, she is returned with the same message: Too old, too damaged!

Frustrated at the lack of cooperation, I lose my composure. As if talking to a child, I tell Bertha in no uncertain terms, "When you leave this goddamn hospital, it's going to be through the front door and on those two legs of yours. Do you understand?"

The whole scene must have been funny. I catch her student nurse trying to suppress something more than a smile.

A month passes. The human deluge continues. Finally, a day comes when, desperately seeking a bed for a new admission, I again realize that of all my patients, the one in the best condition is Bertha Cohen.

With a certain reluctance I now agree to send her off to another ward. Her progress has become an inspiration. As she is about to be wheeled off, I ask, "Where?"

Once again, the answer is, "Rehab."

The rehabilitation ward is a long, rectangular room. The empty bed is at the far end. The student nurse stops the wheelchair about ten feet inside the entrance. I start forward to accompany Bertha on the long journey, only to have the hand of an eighteen-year-old girl catch my arm and hold it fast.

Unspoken are the words, "She is mine!"

The physicians rounding on their patients stop. We all watch Bertha's jerky, awkward movements reduce feet to inches.

They kept her on rehabilitation even when a bed once again became available on our ward.

Yesterday, her student nurse came down to see me. Smiling, she said, "Your sugar-coated bagel, all of seventy-two years, just walked out of Bellevue!"

I can't help hugging her. In another world, when accounts are tabulated, the tribe of Cohen owes one Colleen O'Malley a big one.

## My Lady

In a few minutes the centrifuge will stop. After the urinalysis is completed and the results entered into the chart, it's good night to A-3.

Over three hours ago, p.m. passed into a.m. The lights of the city are naked in their isolation. Suddenly, part of the surrounding darkness comes alive: red lights blinking, an ambulance pulls up to the receiving area. Its silhouette outlines a vehicle too new to be one of ours. This is part of the nightly pilgrimage. Only the names of the ambulances change: Columbia Hospital, Manhattan General, Beckman Downtown, New York Hospital, etc. The message and the contents are almost always the same, "No beds available: send to Bellevue."

For the unwanted and dying, the patients that no other institution wants, deliverance is here.

The chart is complete. There is nothing to do until the new patient is announced. If I'm lucky, she will be admitted to another service, but a little voice tells me she's mine.

Long before my time, one of the wealthy families of New York City had endowed a certain midtown hospital with a pavilion. With this endowment had come an unwritten understanding that when the time arrived, a suite of rooms would always be available to the donors. When that time came for one of the grand-dames of the family, an ambulance was speedily summoned and dispatched. When the admitting resident saw its contents, he hastily conducted a brief physical examination and then wrote: "Sorry, no beds. Please send to Bellevue."

He had not seen a grand-dame in a Bergdorf Goodman gown but an incontinent seventy-nine-year-old female covered with excrement.

Later, when no grand-dame can be found at the midtown hospital, a different form of excrement is dispensed. Finally, in desperation, the hospital's chief of medicine seeks out the night emergency room flow sheet and reads what he most dreads

The family descended upon Bellevue, and the grand-dame was whisked away to her pavilion, where she died five days later in the comfort to which she was accustomed.

The squeak, squeak of the stretcher heralds the arrival of my new patient. The admission sheet reads, "Cerebral vascular accident, old: disposition problem."

In the lower corner in small letters is written, "Sorry."

So at three o'clock in the morning, I take the bony hand of this unwanted human residue in mine and say, "Welcome to Bellevue, my lady."

Her eyes smile back. The light is still on inside.

## Female Medical Clinic

Female medical clinic: two thousand years of anxiety waiting in a room that would depress anybody. The walls are painted a two-tone green that, in all probability, is leftover Army surplus.

Among the patients are those well-advanced along their biological decay curve. They often have no true pathology beyond that anticipated for their age. In the vernacular, they are called *crocks*. At times, the title unquestionably fits.

Today's weekly visit of eighty-two-year-old Sara MacAndrews is different. As always, she is neatly dressed. You can see in her pale blue eyes and carriage the vestiges of what had once been a lovely lady. She doesn't stop with the customary one disease. Somewhere in the midst of the fourth description, I interrupt her and ask, "Sara, what's really wrong?"

She looks at me for a minute, trying to see if I am going to be angry with her, and then she slowly replies, "My sister died two weeks ago."

I almost don't need to ask of what. It has already been described.

At first, I resented these patients diluting the time I have to give to those whose illnesses require more serious medical care. Slowly, I am learning that these ten or fifteen minutes when somebody listens to and is concerned for them is the only real therapy for a disease called loneliness. If untreated, it too kills.

## A Grand Event

It is one of those nights when I am reluctant to leave the ward: just a second sense that something is going to happen.

I check on those who are on the launching pad and then move down to another set of beds. These belong to individuals who are going to die soon and for whom we can offer little but a bed.

When she was well, Misty Butler probably never weighed more than 110 pounds. Now, a combination of cancer and tuberculosis has literally reduced her to skin and bones.

She is special. Even though the end will be soon, there is fire in her big brown eyes. As I pick up her bony hand, her other hand covers mine.

"Don't worry about me. I've been preparing all my life for that day. I was born a sharecropper's daughter, but I will not die as one."

For twenty years, Misty has paid the funeral director five dollars a month.

"It will be a grand event. I will die a lady!"

## When Breath Permits

Four hours ago, seventy-two-year-old Ida Rosenberg began what was probably one of the most terrifying journeys of her life. She had experienced a pain in the left side of her chest for which her memory could find but a single comparable experience.

With the morphine, the pain begins to subside; only she can't breathe. A thousand breaths and still the air hunger between her gasps persists. She tells her neighbor, Mrs. Bloom, in the ambulance, "If I'm to die, they should do it quickly, but not like this."

Mrs. Bloom knows as much about Ida Rosenberg's life as friendship permits—and a bit more. While Ida Rosenberg gurgles for the next breath, Mrs. Bloom does what Mrs. Rosenberg can do only with extreme difficulty: talk! She tells me about the constipation, the ingrown toenail, the rheumatism, the diabetes, and finally about the episodes of chest pain and the heart attack two years previously.

While she talks, I work. She is still talking as she leaves.

The rales that have been up to the apices of her lungs are now receding. Her skin is still clammy, but the purple hue of her skin is beginning to fade. As I start to adjust the oxygen pressure, Ida catches hold of my arm. Removing the face mask, she pulls herself upright in the bed, leans forward from her semi-upright position, and asks without a single pause, "Are you Jewish?"

## Night Becomes Morning

Within my last sixty hours on duty, I've had to helplessly watch three patients die. To hold the hand of dying patients and know there is not a damn thing I can do for them sometimes takes more strength than I now have. They forgot to tell you in medical school that medicine is a game you ultimately lose. It is like the Green Bay Packers playing Nibishville High. If you're good, you will slow them down; but in the end, they carry the ball across—and sometimes a bit of you along with it.

This night, reality and the system that makes these wards the dumping ground for Potter's Field are winning. My thighs ache from standing too long. With a ward full of really sick patients, I know the end of this night's vigil is not near. Standing immobile in the darkness between two beds, looking out the window at the first faint slivers of dawn, I resent a world with the warmth of somebody else beside them. Telling the city what they can do with their twenty cents an hour requires effort. It feels good just not to move.

My thoughts are so concentrated on my fatigue and lack of physical gratification that I am unaware of the old woman in the bed on my right until she takes my hand and kisses it.

In a second, the physical night disappears and the spiritual night becomes morning.

# Part IV

*B4: First Medical Division*

## Matthew Greene

Matthew Greene is forty-nine years old; but the end is near. He has a cruel disease, cancer of the esophagus. The esophagus is a specialized muscular tube connecting the back of the mouth to the stomach. His cancer first impeded the passage of solid food, then semi-liquids, and now the obstruction is almost total. What had been a 189-pound man has turned into a 90-pound skeleton.

He is markedly dehydrated, with a temperature of 104 degrees. This is his fourth admission for pneumonia in the past three months.

Things happen for a reason. In his case, that reason most probably is that his cancer has eroded into the trachea, causing what is called a tracheoesophageal fistula, meaning that the passage for nourishment now connects with that for air. Injecting a blue dye confirms my guess. Material sucked from his windpipe identifies the bacteria involved. After taking appropriate cultures, I hang up a bottle of intravenous fluids containing ten million units of penicillin, confident that his rendezvous with death will be postponed.

Flushed with a certain amount of hubris, which has become my worst enemy, I start to present the case to my resident. He listens, eyes downcast. The quiet anger in his voice cuts me short. He says, "You will cure the infection, but what have you done for the man?"

He walks over to Mr. Greene and takes his hand. They talk. After a few minutes, he reaches up and stops the intravenous fluid infusion. A few minutes later, an emergency room nurse administers morphine. Mr. Greene drops off into a permanent sleep.

## Unanswered Question

I'm still stuck on Matthew Greene. He makes me realize how lucky I am to have had an exceptional teacher like Mara in medical school.

Dr. Mara could have divided the visiting seminary students among all the fourth-year students on the Family Practice rotation. Instead, he chose to proceed differently.

Putting the pipe back into his mouth, he says, "They think that they know people and maybe they do." Then he winks. "But for the next twelve days, I want you to take one of them with you on your house calls."

A theological seminary in Cambridge had requested that their forthcoming graduates participate in the fourth-year medical students' house calls. So a ritual begins, the end of which is almost always the same: the Cottiers.

Mr. Cottier is a retired sergeant from the Royal Canadian Army. When his wife suffered her first cancer, they had just moved to the suburbs of Boston. The second one impoverished them. Now, with her third primary cancer, they are living in the south end of Boston.

She had been cured of the first two, but the third one is different. They have removed her voice box and much more, but the tumor has already spread beyond the margin of tissues that could be surgically removed.

It extends into the confined spaces of the base of the skull. The result is excruciating pain: not a pain that comes and goes, but a pain that is forever constant. I can't decide whether it is fortunate or tragic that she cannot talk.

When I first visit Mrs. Cottier, she is already beyond the help of opiates and almost every combination of drugs. She knows it's the day they change medical students. She is waiting.

As soon as her husband leaves the room, she grabs my arm and presses the note into my hand. As I read it, I have only to glance into her eyes or feel her nails digging into my forearm to understand how real that request is.

With my otoscope, I can see the tumor growing out of the middle ear, but there is nothing I can really do. Her body writhes with pain.

Sometimes alcohol works, sometimes morphine, but those are just short reprieves. All I can really offer is an arm for her to dig her nails into.

Each day for twelve days, outside of the Cottiers' door I turn to someone who, like me, is about to take the vow of a different dedication, and I ask him to give an answer to the request on that piece of paper.

No one does.

Before falling asleep tonight, I more clearly understand that Matthew Greene has been delivered, thanks to someone stronger than me.

## The Front Porch

Just returned from the pastime that I most enjoy—and one I can afford: walking the streets of New York. Downtown, every ten blocks or so a store sells pizza by the slice. The closer you are to Little Italy, the better the pizza.

Something happened today that I can't quite shake out of my memory. If it had been First or Second Avenue, maybe it would not have registered with the same intensity. But it happened on Fifty-Third Street, just off Park Avenue.

A man was lying halfway on the curb, half in the street, convulsing. What I could see of his forehead from across the street told of his previous falls. People moved hurriedly right or left, trying not to look. Some hesitated, looking down in confusion before moving on.

Before the light changed, a young man altered his stride and in slow motion stepped over him and lifted his head. I believed there might be some kind of redemption, until his hand slipped into the man's back pocket.

Maybe it's just New York, but I can't help thinking that what goes around, comes around. Someone once wrote:

*In a world of assembly-line mentalities,*
*men have lost their interdependence and*
*don't care for each other.*

An old farmer from Tennessee whose terminal home is now Bellevue put it more simply. "When they did away with the front porch in America, people lost knowing about and, above all, caring for each other."

## Wrong Direction

In all honesty, the hospital's administration cannot take sole credit for the dilapidated state of this hospital. Too often Bellevue has been funded with crumbs from a very meager budget. What little equipment is bought can all too frequently be found later in the pawn shops on the Lower East Side, courtesy of drug addicts or individuals who just want a little extra chicken for the pot.

During the August heat wave, formaldehyde fumes overcome one of the pathology residents. There is no such thing as air conditioning there. To prevent a reoccurrence, a large exhaust fan is welded into the window. It lasts exactly three days.

Today, I see an orderly pushing a laundry cart filled with laboratory equipment past one of the hospital security guards, who is too engrossed in the *Daily News* to be disturbed. By the time I catch up with the orderly, he is outside the iron front gates.

"I think this is the direction you want to go."

He continues in his direction, and I in mine, a small adjustment having been made.

## Here, Kitty, Kitty

The sub-basements of Bellevue connect via tunnels, remnants from the old Bellevue that burnt down. They are convenient places to store things, in anticipation of a tomorrow that, in the majority of cases, never comes. Sometimes, they harbor broken-down machines from which parts can be salvaged.

The sub-basement is reasonably well-lighted, but its tunnels are not. A journey into Bellevue's underworld requires a good flashlight and a couple of sixty-watt bulbs.

What I need is a two-inch adapter that will connect an endotracheal tube in a patient's throat to a Bird Respirator. Last night, the respirator came, but no adapter. Two inches that could not be breached had separated a life from death.

Finding a tunnel not previously entered, I throw the light switch. Nothing! Change a light bulb. Again, nothing. Opening the fuse box, the reason for the previous failures becomes all too apparent.

Using the flashlight, I carefully make my way through the randomly placed piles of material, searching for Bird Respirators. Flashing my light down the tunnel, a pair of large eyes stares back. My first thought is that a cat has found refuge down here.

The animal does not move as I approach, calling out, "Here, kitty, kitty."

"Here, kitty, kitty" turns out to be about a ten-pound furry animal whose tail has no hair. I am probably the first human this Norwegian rat has ever seen.

For a moment, we just look at each other and then depart in mutually exclusive directions, both convinced that this meeting has lasted too long.

## Proximity's Price

A wide alleyway separates Bellevue Hospital from Bellevue School of Nursing. The passage is much traveled in both directions.

If you desire to see a young lady, you go to the receptionist and identify yourself and the party you wish to see. She then calls the person in question. If the response is positive, you are ushered into a large parlor with comfortable chairs to wait.

The real parlor is Bellevue's public cafeteria. Repeated glances or a smile become your invitation to be interviewed.

The relative commonality of our professional backgrounds, emotional pressures, and physical stress significantly reduces the length of courtships. An unspoken bond of mutual respect provides a foundation for prevailing hormonal imbalances.

But proximity has a price.

Last night, the ward phone rings; the student nurse covering the night shift says, "It's for you."

Debra asks me, "Can I come over?"

Taking great care to imply yes in a conversation that spoke of other topics, I hang up the phone.

The ward is quiet. Unless all hell breaks out, I am not in position to get the next four patients.

A half hour later, the ward having been checked and double-checked, I walk over to the student nurse.

"Call me if anything comes up. I'll be in my room."

About 11:30, I return to the ward.

As I walk by the nurse's station, without looking up, the student nurse asks, "How was it?"

I continued walking as if the question had no significance, until she adds, "That was Debra, wasn't it?"

## Mother by Necessity

The invoice from Cutler Surgical Supplies for the Bird adapter comes to $17.50 plus tax. That is about 17 percent of this month's salary.

The interns working for the City of New York in 1961 have the highest salary in the United States, approximately $1,200 per year, or about $100 per month. At many hospitals, intern and resident pay is so nominal that it is called cigarette money. Why are interns in New York City comparatively better paid? Two years ago, house staff members found out that they qualified for unemployment payments. The City Fathers, in their fiscal wisdom, then raised their pay to a level that would no longer qualify them for unemployment benefits.

Bellevue is more than an institution for learning. By fiscal necessity, she becomes your mother. She houses you, feeds you, clothes you, educates you, and, in a strange way, cares about you. For many of us, affection is a two-way street.

## Second Thoughts

A new 33-rpm disk falls onto the turntable. The voice of Buffy Sainte-Marie replaces that of Joan Baez. Sleep is not far away, which makes the knock on the door both surprising and un-welcome. The tranquility of the moment evaporates.

Reluctantly, I get up off the bed, walk to the door, and open it.

The contrast could have hardly been greater. I am in the doorway dressed in a T-shirt and boxer shorts. The caller is a head shorter, dressed in a three-piece suit. There's no missing the faint scent of cologne.

"Sounds like you're into folk music."

That gets him nowhere. He continues. "You guys must get very lonely. For twenty dollars, you can spend …"

As if scripted, an attractive eighteen- or nineteen-year-old, girl, probably Puerto Rican, moves into the area immediately behind him.

The thought of rearranging his dental alignment or family jewels briefly crosses my mind. The door closes with emphasis. Two steps toward the bed, I stop.

Levi Cohen, one of the NYU interns who lives on the floor, is very smart but forgot to get in line when looks were being passed out. His social life is a negative issue. Once he is in practice, someone will probably exchange bedroom privileges for checking account privileges, but this is now, and we live very much in the now.

The door opens again; I call down the hall. "Try the fourth door down. The name is Levi."

## Chutzpah

In certain instances, an autopsy becomes a legacy that a man leaves his society and his peers. Our patients are the true professors. They are the ones who teach the natural history of a disease.

The head of an orthodox Jewish family died. The case is of considerable importance. To obtain permission for an autopsy from an orthodox family is nearly mission impossible; but it can be done. When you understand why the patient dies, an autopsy is not very critical; but when you work for weeks on a patient and are still baffled at the time of his demise, answers become important.

The problem in this particular case is obvious: Ashton, with his blond hair, blue eyes, and straight nose. His relationship with the family has been great, but that is not going to cut it.

Suddenly, a *deus ex machina* walks through the door in the roly-poly form of Marty Finegold. We used to tease Marty about his corpulence, but he would merely reply, "That comes from too much mother-loving."

Mr. Cantor had been Marty's patient prior to his transfer to another ward. Dramatically snatching the papers out of Ashton's hands, Marty marches up to the relatives who are holding a family council.

"My name is Finegold, as you remember."

He turns his face, giving them a long look at his profile. Turning back he says, "My father is a rabbi. Sign these papers!"

As Marty triumphantly hands Ashton the permission papers, I can't help but rib him. "And what do you call that?"

Looking up over the top of his glasses, he answers, "Chutzpah and a bit of mother-fucking."

## Crashing the Gate

Once winter is here, crashing Bellevue's front gate becomes a struggle for survival. The Bowery fears the winter. There are too few beds available, making dying on the streets a higher probability.

If you're a Bowery resident with an abnormal chest X-ray or you've had tuberculosis, that can potentially be manipulated into hospitalization—until they find out that you are faking. What you do is get a buddy to bleed onto any small piece of white cloth that you can lay your hands on and then claim that you have just coughed up blood. If that doesn't work, you ram a pencil up your urethra so that the urine analysis shows blood in the urine. If that doesn't work, you can try faking total loss of consciousness. Unfortunately, the latter fails when ethyl chloride is sprayed on your genitalia. If that doesn't work, you make a deal with an ambitious surgical resident. He gets an appendix or gallbladder, and you get three to four weeks in a warm bed. And if that doesn't work, you step out in front of a car as it starts up and hope that you live.

Zack Wilson has managed to crash the gate. He has blood in his urine. His breath tells me that he has fortified himself before arranging for his evening accommodations. Once in, he thinks he's on his way to a warm bed and that's it. In the examination room, he passes as close to me as possible. His shoulder brushes mine. His stocky build and posturing says that he is a bully on the streets. Tonight, I am in no mood to deal with an anal-aggressive alcoholic.

His medical history, present illness, and review of systems having been done, the physical examination is next.

"Mr. Wilson, please take off your clothes."

"It's late, doc, and I'm tired," comes the reply. His hands make no move toward his sweater or pants. The request is repeated, but now without the *please*. Nothing!

I turn to the evening nurse. "Call security and have them throw him out on the street."

Her facial expression says *I don't believe this!* She timidly answers, "Are you sure?"

Never taking my eyes off the patient, I reply with an emphatic, "Yes!"

She dials the first two numbers. The sweater comes off, then the shirt, then the shoes and socks, and finally the pants. This is where I usually ask the nurse to leave. Not tonight.

"Okay?" he asks. Defiance is still there but now more subdued.

"Everything!"

After a long moment, a dirty undershirt and underpants join his other clothes. He stands completely naked, illuminated by the focused light from the high-intensity examination lamp. The long silence intensifies his nakedness.

"If, after the examination is over, I find that you are really sick, I will do everything in my power to make you well. If you're uncomfortable with that, tomorrow morning ask for another doctor. Do we have a clear understanding?"

There is no defiance in the answer.

"Kathy, you can now put the phone down. Please let me have the room."

A physical examination reveals a recently dilated urethra with a small amount of bright red blood coming out. Percussion over the kidneys does not demonstrate the presence of underlying tenderness. The blood work is fine.

When the examination is through, I ask, "Pencil or screw driver?"

The curt answer: "Neither. A fountain pen with its point bent."

For the first time this evening, we are on the same page.

Once Mr. Wilson is settled into Hotel Bellevue for his three-day stay, Kathy comes up to me. "That was ugly. I almost have a mind to report your conduct."

Kathy's right. I came dangerously close to abrogating the patient/doctor relationship. But for it to exist, both must want it.

## Little Words

Language is meant for communication. Once again, big words were used when little words were needed.

Nowhere in medical school is the art of patient communication taught. In the service of a two-year-old boy, Stevie Fallow, I first learned the power of little words.

They were shorthanded in pediatrics at the Boston City Hospital. My then girlfriend being in Europe, I volunteered to do my fourth-year pediatric rotation in the capacity of an intern.

Stevie was one of the patients I inherited. His condition required that I take blood for analysis every other day. What should have been a barrier became a bond between us. The relationship developed to the point where I would ask and he would hold out his arm for the needle and syringe. Through Stevie I got to know the family, especially his father, Malco Fallow.

Stevie's father had waged the battle of Warsaw and lost. Mutilated, with only one arm and one eye, he had worked in France until he could pay for passage to the United States for his wife and four children. Getta, the oldest child, had told me with pride how upon disembarking in America, her father had told them, "We may never be rich, but there is one thing I promise you ... there'll always be food in the house."

One had only to look at Mrs. Fallow and the children to understand how well he had kept that promise. He worked as a janitor in one of the elementary schools in South Boston during the day and pumped gas at a filling station in Newton at night. Little by little, the Fallows acquired those material things that help to embellish life.

Stevie was the gift of the Promised Land: silver blond hair, fair complexion, and blue eyes, to which was added a photogenic beauty that went beyond being a two-year-old. Then one day, Stevie began losing weight. His abdomen began to swell, and little red spots appeared on his body.

Malco Fallow took Stevie not to the local clinic which would have been free, but to the best hospital in Boston. When asked if he could pay, Malco Fallow answered, "Sure I pay! You just make my son well."

When the bill came from Children's Hospital, Malco Fallow said not a word. He went to his bank. Two days later, men came in a truck to pick up some of the furniture. The Fallows were materially poorer. It did not matter. Stevie was back. But he was not well. He had been discharged with the diagnosis of meningococcemia, an invasion of the bloodstream by a specific type of bacteria. Now two months later, the diagnosis was evident. Stevie had an acute form of leukemia. He would likely be dead in the next three to four months.

Malco Fallow could not accept that his son's deterioration was due an incurable disease. He saw in the dirt and neglect of a big-city hospital the rationale to attribute Stevie's downhill course to something else. When Getta told Catherine, the co-intern, and me that more furniture had been sold, we both knew that it was only a question of time before Malco would go again in search of a magic mountain.

I had just finished a white blood cell count when Cathy burst in.

"He did it! He just picked Stevie up and left! Will you come?"

The Fallows live in Class C housing, but their house stands out from the rest. Getta is waiting for us. She knows we are coming. Despite being only eleven years-old, she understands all too well the selling of the furniture.

Mrs. Fallow and the rest of the children meet us in the front room.

Stevie has been my responsibility. I begin, only to find that I am speaking in a language intelligible in the coffee houses of Harvard Square but impotent in this situation.

Cathy takes over. For the next ten minutes, I listen to a vocabulary so simple, yet poignant. Mrs. Fallow asks, "Any hope?"

Cathy answers, "A little," as she holds her thumb and index finger half an inch apart and slowly brings them together.

Mrs. Fallow begins crying. Turning her tear-stained face upward, she says, "I give you Stevie, but Malco …"

He had seen the car and knew why we were there. Despite his wiry five-foot-six frame and angular build, there was nothing diminutive about him. From the moment he enters through the door, you know that this is his home.

Cathy starts, but Malco Fallow is not going to have a woman tell him what to do. They have a place, but it is not in front of him.

Without my wanting it, the talking stick is back in my hand. Eyes fixed to eyes, I speak slowly, using small, carefully chosen words whose force I have just witnessed. It takes a while to master their power. When I feel it, I go for Stevie. It is hard to tell a loving father that he needs to release the dying to save the living.

Finally, Malco turns his face away from me, so that what he is now ready to accept is heard but not seen. "You take Stevie. God damn you if you don't take good care of him!"

Mrs. Fallow and Getta walk the three of us back to the car.

The day Stevie Fallow died, I am sure Malco Fallow cursed my name; but that is a small price to pay for the gift Stevie left with me. Tomorrow, I am going to need those little words.

## Sooner

His arrival at Bellevue was logical. His Lincoln Continental had been involved in a multi-vehicle accident on First Avenue, three blocks away. John Quinn's stay on the public wards of Bellevue Hospital was not.

In the emergency room, a history of progressive double vision, intense head pain, and blacking out is elicited. Because he's a member of the board of one of New York's most powerful financial institutions, he's offered an immediate transfer to a private institution. The offer is declined.

In the course of doing his review on the ward, a little different history is obtained: changes in bowel habits and the recent onset of occasional episodes of crampy abdominal pain. The test for blood in the stool is positive.

His physical appearance and reputation are dipoles apart: a short man with wavy white hair and deep blue eyes framed by horn-rimmed glasses. In a larger body frame, he could have been a perfect Santa Claus. What makes it all work is a smile that forces you to respond in kind.

He is my last patient. The initial workup takes longer than usual, owing to tangential conversations that ventured into nonmedical realms.

Neurology consultants from both Cornell Medical Center and Presbyterian Hospital do John Quinn's initial workup. He is transported uptown in the morning and returned in the early evening. The nights when I am on service and the ward is quiet, we talk about many things, until one night, without being asked, he revealed why Bellevue.

Our conversations have always been honest, but tonight it becomes brutally honest. He tells of having been a big-time drinker. Alcohol lost him his wife, his two daughters, and almost his life.

With great difficulty, he talks about what made him the man he is today: his daughter who died of pneumonia because there was no money in the house for the cab.

Why Bellevue? "I have walked in their shoes. Service with gratitude is what allowed me to make it beyond one day at a time. Until you get there, you're nothing but a dry drunk faking it.

"My higher power put me here so that I might see about doing something in the time remaining for others who are here and who suffer from the same disease."

He knows!

Once the neurological diagnosis of an intracranial mass is arrived at through consensus, the downtown workup begins in earnest. The finding of blood in his stool is the reason for a sigmoidoscopy.

The instrument goes in thirteen inches. There is no need to go further. What is needed is a biopsy. The abnormal liver function tests are the reason for the second biopsy.

The next morning, the biopsy reports are in the chart. The diagnosis in the chart is now "poorly differentiated adenocarcinoma of the bowel metastatic to brain and liver." There is no thread of hope to cushion the statement's finality.

Since his arrival, the ritual during morning attending rounds is always the same: an occult nod of the head to signify acknowledgement until we reach his bedside. This morning, the nod is forced.

Once it is his turn to be seen on attending rounds, the words are short and simple.

Taking his right hand in mine, I tell him, "Bill, God wants you home sooner than we thought."

His grip on my hand tightens.

## New Year's Eve

The room is empty. Scattered paper cups and two empty bottles of champagne say that New Year's has come and gone. A full glass and a note from Marvin are on the table. What has kept me away has claimed the others. Three small bubbles valiantly cling to the bottom of the glass. It's too late for Chicago and too early for Denver. Everything is a couple of light years removed from a year ago in Boston. Yet, the fact that with this day I will have survived six months makes New Year's worth celebrating.

## A Different Bed

As an intern at Bellevue, there are two places you can sleep in a bed: your bedroom and the ward.

If no night nurse is available and you have a critically ill patient, a cot is put next to his or her bed. With luck, you get to use it.

But that is not the only reason one goes under the sheets on the ward.

We almost always have one or two addicts on a male ward: usually for viral hepatitis, drug dependency withdrawal, or drug overdose. Most of the addicts who come in for withdrawal are not seeking freedom from addiction. Their habit has gotten too expensive.

Bellevue Hospital is anything but a drug-free environment. If you want a hamburger, a beer, or heroin, you can get it. After spending several weeks bringing patients to the edge of being drug-free, they sign out AMA: against medical advice. Nothing has changed, except the amount of drug needed to get high.

Willie McCord's withdrawal is nearly complete. This is when the pusher sends in the test sample. Tonight, Tom, my resident, and I will be waiting for the goodie man to arrive— not in the beds, under them.

The schedule has been altered so that no night nurse will be on duty. Willie McCord is given sleeping pills with his medications.

About one o'clock, the ward telephone rings and goes unanswered. Presuming that someone is checking, we quietly take our positions.

We don't have to wait long. A flashlight beam systematically checks the beds on both sides to make certain that patients are patients. Soon two thick white socks are twenty inches from my face.

"Hey, man. Wake up! Do you want it or not?"

Tom answers for him. "No, he doesn't!"

Thrusting both legs out sideways from under the bed, I kick out both his ankles. Before he can recover, a heavy flashlight and a knee in the small of his back convince him not to move.

This should have been hospital security's job. But security, like this porter, is part of the permanent staff.

## Miss PanAm

There is something about death that ignites primitive instincts for survival of the species.

When interns rotate off one ward to another, bonds of dependency are broken. Patients, particularly those without much family, often come to rely on the daily contacts for reassurance of a maybe tomorrow. Sometimes, these are their last ties to life. When disrupted, the light within sometimes goes out.

The rotation brings me back again to A-3. It's Monday.

Tuesday holds the promise of being a good day. The ward has the rare complement of two RNs: our ward nurse and a PanAmerican stewardess who needs to work one day a month to keep her nursing certificate valid. The occasional extra nurse is payment for my not visiting the hospital administrator.

The first patient literally codes during morning attending physician's rounds. Despite everyone's best efforts, she is pronounced dead at 7:37 a.m.

In the afternoon, code number two occurs.

The crisis of the moment swallows time. Before we can take a deep breath and sense the joy of accomplishment with code number two, a third patient codes, and twenty minutes later, the patient in the bed to her right codes.

No time to change the position of the curtains around the bed or to get a board under her. The bed to the left is pushed against the adjacent bed. A firm foundation is needed to do CPR; she is quickly put on the floor. A tube is inserted into her windpipe. Two intravenous fluid lines are started, and her heart is manually stimulated by compression.

After the second code, the medical student, nursing student, Miss PanAm, and I achieve fluidity. The need to ask for something vanishes. My hand goes out and returns with what is needed.

Not until the night shift intern moves me over do I realize the hour. A new team is taking over. Three of the patients who coded had belonged to the other team. Mine had died that morning. The patient on the floor is alive, but barely. She might make it through the night, but anything more is in God's hands.

It is now past 6:00 p.m., an hour past the change of interns for the night, but three hours past the time when Miss Pan Am could have left the ward.

For maybe the first time, I take a really hard look at her: Irish, flaming bright red hair, blue eyes, and freckles. Definitely good-looking.

As we walk off the ward and down the corridor, her hand seeks mine and finds an answer forged by a mutual desire to escape the shadows of death just departed.

## The Cup

Dr. Hauser has been the ward's attending physician. Now that his month has come to an end, the B-4 interns and residents find us in the back room of the White Horse Tavern, commemorating the parting of ways.

Probably for the first time since the death of his wife, Dr. Hauser has unleashed the burden of sobriety. Somewhere in the beer and bourbon, the physician is absolved and the poet reborn.

What is first said in light-hearted jest takes on a different tone. Brandishing his stein aloft, his eyes like lights in reflecting pools, he recites:

> "I heard a voice within the tavern cry,
> Awake, my little ones and fill the Cup
> Before Life's liquor in its Cup be dry."

The hurt is still there. He tries to start another stanza, only to falter. Suddenly, tired of the game, he cuts himself short. Though drunk, his voice takes on that earnest intensity we have learned to appreciate in the month just passed.

"Being a physician, you will learn much about life. By their needs, your patients will become your teachers. In their hour of greatest need, they will stand before you … naked! It is this recognition and its sharing that will permit you to be taught beyond your years. It takes a very blunt mind not to see and understand how often we come to death with thirsting lips, the Cup having long been dry. Not having comprehended that, we die wretched little deaths."

The tone of his voice gains body. "But among the many, there are a few who in the face of death reveal that rare thing called dignity."

His voice begins to crack and the words slur. "Once you've met one, you will understand the legacy they leave us, the living."

Head on the table, subdued in his thoughts, he is reunited with the person who had shared his life.

## Snow

The first heavy snow of the year is gently falling. Walking back from the Village, I now pass individuals whom I have seen on my way downtown. But this time, they are out of their territory.

The big push for a nickel or dime is on. After a Boweryite hits you up, you can barely count to ten before he disappears into a local package store. But tonight, there is a difference. They really mean it when they ask you for it.

When a car stops at a red light, at least two of them run up and begin cleaning the windows with dirty rags or their undershirts. There is probably not a nickel slot in any local telephone booth that hasn't been gummed.

When I walk into the reception area, they are already massing. I guess there are about two hundred men and a handful of women. They are sitting or lying on the benches, leaning against the two-tone green walls, or just standing around. Torn army jackets, pants too big, shoes that don't match, a motley assortment of clothes, tonight unified by something else.

One of the NYU residents clues me in. The year before, there had been a very heavy snowfall. The city had to pull interns temporarily off service to ride the ambulances. When the snow receded, they found several hundred of them in the doorways or on the pavements where they had first fallen in drunken slumber, remaining there until they were no more.

I recognize one of them as once having been my patient.

"Zack, what's the matter?"

"They're scared."

"Why?"

"The snow and the …."

"And you?"

"Look, doc, can you get me in?" And then, perhaps for the first time in our relationship: "Please?"

## A Drop of Truth

There was a time when being a doctor meant something. The breakdown of the traditional doctor-patient relationship has isolated patient and doctor from each other. Like any mutual disassociation, there are two losers. Without a doctor-patient relationship, both are uncommitted.

The tragedy of this is not apparent until somebody needs a physician and goes shopping. In the absence of a true emergency, the good ones are not going to take you on. They have already made their commitments. To protect obligations, they must say no. In time of need, a person is freefalling with respect to competence.

I am at a cocktail party listening to the gory consequences of just such a disfranchisement, when a cute blonde slips her arm around my waist and asks, "And what do you do?"

Cute, but not that cute. Half in jest, I answer, "I'm a sanitation engineer."

Expressive gold-green eyes cloud with confusion.

"A what?" she responds.

"Garbage collector," I reply.

From society's point of view, there is a just drop of truth in that statement.

What is the world record for a heel-spin?

## Reflections of the Father

Your peers are as much your teachers as your patients.

Bob Tate came from the westernmost part of West Virginia. When he was fourteen, his minister father died in a mining accident while administering last rights. Bob put himself through Penn State. He graduated near the top of his class from the University of Pennsylvania College of Medicine. Bob claims to be an agnostic. But his reasons for being a doctor stem from stuff that had led his father to minister in the mines.

His father had been born in England. He had spent his early life among books and ultimately obtained a librarian's degree. The loss of both parents brought him to the United States. There was little work for a foreign librarian. The Eastman Kodak people in Rochester, New York, took him on as an apprentice. They must have wondered what a trained librarian was doing among their machine shop applicants. Ultimately, he became a lens press operator. He had to press lenses eight hours a day. The work was empty of any objective purpose.

He never abandoned his love for books and nearly always carried a copy of the New Testament in his pocket. One day, standing in the pay-line, he came across a passage in the New Testament that captured his attention: *"In whatever you do in word or deed, do all in the name of the Lord Jesus and give thanks to God the Father by Him."*

He wondered if this applied to him and his machine. He tried it. The ennui that he had felt at the workbench disappeared. He did so well that he was promoted to the position of a specialist. When Mr. Eastman wanted a special camera, he was the individual chosen to stamp the lens. He became the master of his machine and, in time, invented a number of improvements that, in turn, greatly advanced his professional status. He had more time to study the Bible, until a day arrived when he understood the direction of his personal journey. That principle learned in the machine shop is also ingrained in Bob.

Three weeks ago, Bob began waking up nightly in a drenching sweat. When he discovered that he had a fever, he read more significance into the cold that just didn't seem to clear up. An X-ray revealed a right upper lobe infiltrated with early cavitation. He has tuberculosis. Exactly which patient he got it from, he will never be sure. Approximately 5 percent of the admissions to Bellevue have or have had active pulmonary tuberculosis.

If he is lucky, it'll be a year before he can again be admitted into an internship. While his hometown banker will wait for repayment of the principal on the loans, the interest payments will not wait.

As he walks, suitcase in hand, past a group of orderlies, I hear one of them remark, "Maybe when he comes back he'll be less of an all-American Boy Scout."

## Not Bricks

Dr. Salvatore Cutolo has practiced medicine for over forty years. He has worked at Bellevue in the capacity of deputy medical administrator for thirty-six of those years. But now his position carries little authority. An old man with carefully combed white hair, stooped shoulders, and a rounded back, which his age (and osteoporosis) imposes, he moves with a shuffled walk. He is given great respect. No one dares to suggest that he retire. That would be an unwarranted death sentence.

He is devoted to this antiquated, rat-infested institution. The inadequacies of the hospital described to him don't seem to register. The myths surrounding this institution have partially blinded him to what modern technology can provide.

In our talks, his replies are not always answers but a sometimes tangential recounting of the great men he has known, his "wizards of medicine": DuBois, Sayer, Welch, Richardson …

In the midst of one such exchange between youth and age, he notes my appreciative stare at the large, framed photograph of Bellevue Hospital hanging over his office desk.

Slowly turning around he says, "She's not much to look at, but then; Bellevue is not a story of bricks or technology, is she? Bellevue is a tale of men and women!"

Today, a large, mounted copy of that same photograph is delivered to the ward, signed "With my best wishes. Sincerely, Salvatore Cutolo."

## Ashes to Ashes

Abel Friedman is far from being a nobody. Until his strokes, he has been a major player on Wall Street. Why he is here in Bellevue is not immediately evident.

A son-in-law in California has given me the name of a lawyer and undertaker to contact once he's dead. His other daughter in New Jersey has a pressing social engagement—a charity event. His nephews ask me to keep them informed.

I return to his bedside. The rabbi sits there a while longer, until he too has somewhere else to go.

It is said that you are immortal as long as you are loved and remembered; thereafter, it doesn't matter.

Dust to dust, ashes to ashes is here a little early for Abel Friedman.

## A Matter of Pennies

At 3:00 a.m. last night, I had the dubious honor of getting the first patient. Thomas Keith, a comatose, unresponsive white male is admitted to the emergency room. He had been found unconscious in a doorway. It isn't long before the second and third such cases roll through the doors.

Thomas Keith died a little before 11:00 a.m, but already cases numbers five and six have been admitted. They are all derelicts with no permanent address who have been found in the street, in doorways, or in two-bit flop houses.

Keith's body is immediately transported to the medical examiner's building. By 2:30 p.m., we have confirmation of what had been our clinical impression: methyl alcohol toxicity. Even before his autopsy is finished, the second such admission is already in the hallway of the mortuary.

By the time we get back, it is evident the word is out. Information and rumors normally travel fast in the Bowery, but fear gives them wings.

The admission room is already clogged with the vanguard of what will be 1,100 Boweryites seeking admission. Within seventy-two hours, nine others have died, either on the streets or at Bellevue, Columbia, or the Beekman Downtown Hospital, the traditional addresses of men who have lost their identity.

.    The first patients admitted had been comatose. Within forty-eight hours after admission, they had all died. The second group came in with liver failure. From them, fragments of a story begin to form. In lucid moments, they tell of consuming what they thought to be good alcohol from cans during a curbside drinking bout. What separates them from their dead comrades is the quantity consumed. Search of the Men's Municipal Shelter at 8 East Third Street yields several empty cans of a paint solvent called Elmesco. Elmesco sells for about forty-five cents a pint and can be bought in hardware stores on Sundays when the bars are closed.

Most of those who provided the initial leads lapsed into a coma or died before they could clarify their story. Nevertheless, we now have the how, but not all of the whys. Normally, the percent of methyl alcohol in paint thinner is between 3 and 5 percent. Because methyl alcohol is cheaper than ethyl alcohol, increasing the percentage beyond this limit saves money. The Elmesco that had been consumed had a methyl alcohol content of 80 percent. It had been further cut with cheap hydrocarbons.

May 9: death toll from methyl alcohol poisoning reaches thirty-one. One out of every four medical beds is now being used exclusively for this catastrophe. But now we are seeing fewer patients admitted with liver failure and more with kidney failure. These are primarily the "white smoke" drinkers, those who squeezed alcohol from jelly sterno, or "canned heat," and mixed it with water or 7-Up soda. The methyl alcohol in these products has built up a degree of tolerance that allows them to survive the immediate sequelae of methyl alcohol ingestion.

May 12: the fortieth Boweryite died today. May 13: death toll is forty-four. On May 14, the death toll has risen to forty-eight.

It's pretty much now over. More than sixty-three men and two women have died, primarily of methyl alcohol poisoning. I don't know how many more are left permanently blind or with severe worsening of their liver disease. Two hundred and seventy-three human beings are returned from Bellevue to the Bowery.

The whys: The individuals who bootlegged cheap wine to the Bowery on Sunday had upped the price of a pint from fifty to seventy-five cents. It's more than the local economy can handle. On the third weekend of relative abstinence, the word comes: the paint solvent Elmesco can be cut and drunk. Only one problem—somewhere along the line, the paint thinner formula has been altered. On Sunday, the First of May party becomes a massacre in which a quest for pennies is paid for in lives.

## Score: Country One

The exchanges between our new attending for the month and Chet Hoffermeir are getting to be more and more intense. Chet had owned a farm about thirty miles from Jackson, Tennessee. When bad times came, the bank took his farm, the Bowery took his dignity, and now cancer has a mortgage on his life. Until a nursing home bed for his terminal illness can be found, B-4 remains his only residence.

Having been sober now for months, Chet does his darnedest to find purpose for the time remaining. He has a great sense of humor. When the mood moves him, he embellishes rounds with a version of "how we do it in the country."

Our new attending is all business and good at it. He has no time for banter. His attitude toward Chet is, basically, "This patient is going to die, so let us move on to others, where intervention matters."

Whether it is to preserve those minutes of human contact or not, a new topic has been interjected into morning rounds: more specifically, the origins of certain night sounds. Chet claims rats. Our attending, who lives in Scarsdale, contends that Chet is delusional. Once the argument is initiated, attending morning rounds at his bedside lose their brevity. Both of them have become obsessed with prevailing.

Strangely, today there's no mention of night sounds. We are about to go to the next bed, when Chet casually says to our attending, "Doctor, I have a present for you to take home."

With that, he dramatically throws his bed cover back toward the foot of the bed. The bodies of three very dead rats grace the underlying sheet.

Score: country one/city zero.

## Barton & Sons

Making the turnoff from Sutton Place, you can find Barton & Sons, a small, exclusive tailor shop specializing in custom-fitted suits. Maybe it's a steady diet of second-hand clothes chosen for utility rather than looks that makes that bolt of herring-bone tweed look so good. On my third or fourth trip past Barton & Sons, I stop and go in.

It's immediately apparent that my dress is not that of their usual customers. After a long wait, one of the two sales persons comes over, inquiring as to how he can help me out. The trappings of wealth make me a little self-conscious. I wonder if the words *help* and *out* might have some added significance.

I inquire as to the cost of a suit. Without a hesitation comes the response, "One hundred and fifty dollars, if done in one fitting."

From the way he says it, he anticipates a quick termination to our discussion. Just then, the older clerk, having just finished with a client, comes over. "I'll take care of the gentleman, James."

He immediately walks over to the front display window and carefully lifts the bolt of tweed out. Walking toward me, he says, "It's really a beautiful piece of material."

I am surprised that he knows precisely what has caught my fancy, until he adds, "I've seen you on several occasions admiring it in the window. I'm Mr. Barton of Barton & Sons."

When we are through, an agreement is reached. After five monthly payments of $12.50, I will come in and be measured. After five additional payments, the suit will depart with me. The internship will be over before that suit is ever paid off.

The desire of possession now gives direction to my walks in a certain part of New York.

## Mayhem

The patient's right flank has just been cleansed with an iodine and alcohol solution and the liver biopsy tray is open when the page comes over the loudspeaker system: "Mayhem—A-4, Mayhem. ***Stat!***"

Off come the surgical gloves. *Shame to waste a sterile biopsy tray!*

Running at full speed down the short hall connecting B-4 and A-4, I pass two security guards coming up the middle stairs. Turning left into the A-4 corridor, the reason for "Mayhem" becomes obvious.

I arrive just in time to see Samuel Brown launch the treatment cart through the air. The small handwashing sink at the front of the ward has been partially torn from the wall.

Water spurts in pulses over the floor from a ruptured pipe. To the far left of the door is a motionless pair of legs in white pants. Down at the very far end of the ward, the ward nurse has gathered her nurse's aides around her.

Samuel Brown is a truck driver with arms that resemble small tree trunks attached to a 275-pound body. After twenty years of heavy binge drinking, his liver and brain have teamed up to conjure up things far more frightening than little pink elephants. He is in full-blown DTs: delirium tremens. As he is demonstrating with frightening proficiency, individuals in the DTs can have extraordinary strength.

Terrified by the demons of his illusions, he has snapped his restraints and is now lashing out at what only he can see.

His back is to me. Having played football in high school and knowing that reinforcements are apparently some twenty yards behind me, my decision is easy.

Literally sliding the last five feet, my arms wrap themselves around Samuel Brown's ankles. I lift them to my chest. Samuel Brown's massive frame hits the ground with a resounding thud. The fall momentarily stuns Mr. Brown. That gives me the opportunity to scale his back and get my arms under Samuel Brown's arms and then back around his neck, a position otherwise known in wrestling as a full nelson.

Normally, a full nelson gives you control over someone, but not when that someone has a size eighteen neck and outweighs you by more than a hundred pounds. As he arches his neck and back, my wet fingers begin slipping apart. By shifting my body weight perpendicular to Samuel Brown's body, I gain a very brief advantage. I need help and need it now!

Looking over my shoulder, I see the two security guards timidly peeking in from where the ward meets the corridor.

In response to "Get the hell in here!" comes "Doc, I'm not sure we are authorized to get involved."

That's bullshit! I had witnessed a number of occasions when security physically decimated some poor undersized son of a bitch after he resisted. Apparently, size does matter.

Now my predicament is getting more serious by the millisecond. The full nelson is now a half nelson and soon to be a no nelson. Looking back at the unconscious form at the front of the ward, I know the worse is yet to come.

"Can I help?" inquires a calm, serene voice

Standing over us is eighty-four-year-old Thomas J. Thorten, a one-time writer for the *New Yorker*. Without waiting for an answer, he lifts a heavy metal bed pan with both hands. The sound of metal meeting skull resonates in my ears. Two more mighty love taps and Mr. Brown becomes still.

Normally, my first reaction would be either to thank Mr. Thorten for probably saving my life or to tend to Mr. Brown, who hopefully only has a very bad concussion. But at this moment, neither is foremost on my priority list.

The security guards are now running with full knowledge that they are in harm's way. The bedpan has a new master!

## Bellevue Nurses

When Dr. Cutolo says Bellevue is the story of its men and women, under the heading of *women* there should be a special notation for Bellevue's ward nurses. They are graduates of America's first nursing school, a school founded upon the principles of Florence Nightingale.

Being a ward nurse at Bellevue Hospital is a title of nobility for which there is little or no recognition. As physicians, we make the diagnosis, but it is the ward nurse who converts words into healing.

Just about every ward nurse here wears a Bellevue School of Nursing cap. Each year, a number of them steps forward from each graduating class and take on a challenge that few men would even contemplate: thirty-two beds, filled with a primarily geriatric population for which they dispense all medication, do or oversee all nursing care, do physicians' rounds, and then change the sheets when accidents occur when the nurse's aides are on breaks. She or an aide will have just gotten through going down a row of beds when the need arises to start all over again.

They are among the gutsiest women I will ever meet. After two to three years, they tend to burn out and then take positions at prestigious private hospitals for much higher pay. New ones step forward and take their places.

Having spent the better part of my medical residency on A-3, I place its ward nurse on a pedestal. Among the nurses, she and one of the Cornell nurses are considered the best. But as a Bellevue nurse, her position on the pedestal has added cachet.

## Moses

Internship and residency are strange hybrids, between employment and apprenticeship. At the turn of the century, an individual wishing to become a physician would apprentice himself to a physician for a prescribed period of time. Compensation for his services primarily consisted of the knowledge that he derived.

Somehow, a form of this type of indentured servitude has persisted into the twentieth century. In the past, becoming a physician almost required you to be from a moneyed background. Not infrequently, physicians-to-be were the sons of physicians. It was and still is presumed that if you apply for an internship, you have the means to support yourself.

After World War II, the growing complexity and diversification of medicine expanded medical training from one to two years, or in some cases seven years, of postgraduate training. The GI Bill expanded the pool of qualified candidates. To specialize, you will have completed an approved internship and residency program and passed a national qualifying examination. With an expanding candidate pool competing for a finite number of programs, hospitals took advantage of the concept inherent in the apprenticeship model, in which service is exchanged for learning: the assumption is that the "apprentice/intern/resident" will make up the financial deficit in time.

Working a hundred or more hours a week is not uncommon at large municipal hospitals. This is an injustice that will not self-heal.

The year before I came to Bellevue, the revolt had started. A couple of hundred residents, primarily from King's County Hospital in Brooklyn and Bellevue, got together to discuss forming a union. Apparently, somebody's father was a fire chief or something like that. One way or another, the group ended up in the office of the attorney for the City of New York's Fireman's and Policeman's Benevolence Association. If you are a New York politician and want to remain one, he is one person that you don't piss off.

The story goes that after hearing their story, the attorney told the hundred or so interns and residents to go down to the building's lobby and elect a president, vice president, secretary, and treasurer. Those four individuals, and only those four individuals, were to come back upstairs and discuss the formation of the Intern's and Resident's Committee as the bargaining entity for all house staff members employed by the City of New York.

In that meeting, an agreement was reached that fifty cents of every house staff's paycheck would be paid to his firm from any and all contracts negotiated by him with the City of New York on the committee's behalf.

Now more than a year later, the house staff representatives from the major hospitals sit in oversized red leather chairs within the mahogany-paneled conference room, waiting to hear the results of the just-completed contract.

Primarily by default, I am the vice president of the Bellevue committee. I have mixed feelings about the whole issue. My father would flip if he knew what I am doing. For him, unionism and professionalism are ultimately incompatible. In his mind, the nobility of unionism usually deteriorates into a defense of mediocrity. But I can't see that as being true for medicine. As long as a patient-doctor relationship exists and nothing or no one gets in between, we'll be okay. But God help us all if that ever changes.

The pronouncement that we will be receiving $200 a year more in each of the next two years meets with near silence. Most present are hoping for a *deus ex machina* to lighten their debt burdens. Four years of college, four years of medical school, and three to seven years of internship and residency are a long time to go without a significant pay check.

I know that Jack will take the news badly. He does. Jack had come to medicine via the GI Bill. He is older than the rest of us: married with two kids, one of whom is now seriously ill. He had hoped that the pay increase would allow his wife to stay home with his daughter.

He gets up. I expect him to explode in a burst of anger and frustration. Somehow, he regains his composure. In a voice that betrays disappointment and then something more, he gets up, saying, "I have to leave."

He does so abruptly. Copies of the agreement are handed out. The meeting quickly breaks up.

I stay seated in my chair. Apparently, the lawyer anticipated another type of response. The two or three thank-yous are weak. His face is sober—a far cry from the joking demeanor with which he had started the meeting.

He starts talking. I'm not quite sure if my presence is necessary. "You rich kids were nothing; less than 1 percent of all the house staff employed by the City of New York. I made you the bargaining group for the whole fucking bunch. Before unions there was no real democracy, just masters and fiscal slaves."

Now specifically acknowledging my continued presence, he continues. "Yeah, the first contract isn't much; but it was one the City could easily swallow." His fist comes down emphatically on the table. "The next time we negotiate, they are going to choke!"

The tone is resolute but bittersweet.

His voice now fills with passion. "Your kind is probably too obtuse to understand, but today we have made history. What has happened in New York will reset the employment standards for every intern and resident in the United States."

He pauses. "Two years from now, your bonds of servitude will be forever changed."

This meeting is now truly over. I get up and shake his hand. Unsure of how he will take it, I wait until I'm one step away from the door. As I pass through the conference room's large doors, I turn and say in a loud voice, "Thank you, Moses."

## The Rock

For Kahlil Amourian, life stopped on a mountain in Turkey. He and his family had been part of a bloody episode in history. Men from that part of the world carry a unique definition. They are rocks, the end products of the brutal process of natural selection in which their very existence becomes an enigma to adversity and disease. Most of them have never known what it is to be seriously ill. While death is the common denominator of life, it is almost a foreign concept for them to comprehend emotionally. When a rock tells you that he has a little pain in his chest, you understand that he is telling you about something that would have caused most of us to break the bonds of silence.

When he descended the other side of the mountain, he left behind the warm corpses that had been his life. For him, existence becomes hard work and the simple pleasures that he permits. He is a builder with nothing or no one to build for. He dwells in a realm of emotional and material self-reliance until the day, somewhere in his seventies, when he begins to notice the onset of a hacking nocturnal cough. At night, he finds it necessary to prop himself up in bed with two pillows. Then, the night comes when two pillows fail and he has to spend it standing at the window. Finally a night comes when even that does not suffice. He cannot breathe. A single breath comes so hard. In the early morning hours, years of self-reliance crumble. Blue, cyanotic, gasping for breath, his pajamas wet with perspiration, for the first time in his life, Kahlil Amourian needs someone else's strength.

At 4:00 a.m., Kahlil Amourian is admitted to the emergency room. In the first few hours many procedures happen to him: oxygen, drugs to dilate his air passages, drugs to strengthen his heart, drugs to rid his body of excess water. There is a moment when Kahlil Amourian is more concerned about losing his pants than his breath; but his helplessness in the face of his disease ultimately compels him to accept the hospital nightshirt. While we fight to bring his disease to bay, another battle is periodically waged. Ten times or more the oxygen mask hits the emergency floor. To be sick is one thing, but to have physical evidence of his infirmity strapped to his face is more than he apparently intends to tolerate. By 7:00 a.m., he gets reprieve. By noon, anxiety and disease have given way to sleep.

That night, Kahlil Amourian is transferred to an up-ward. The next day his lungs are clear. The small patch of fine rales in the posterior gutter has now totally disappeared. His pulse rate is normal. His heartbeat is regular. His cardiogram shows an enlarged left side of the heart, but no evidence of recent damage. If he maintains his present course, barring complications, in the months to come he will have his diseased aortic valve replaced. If successful, this operation will significantly prolong his life.

There is just one thing wrong: Kahlil Amourian. The hands that had wrenched the oxygen mask from mine are limp. His eyes hold a nebulous, glassy stare.

On evening rounds as I tell my cointern about my patients, their therapy, and their anticipated complications, the sight of his massive weather-beaten frame is disturbing. His shoulders sag, but what is really upsetting is that he remains in virtually the same position as during morning rounds.

When I get to my room, I go through the ritual performed so often these past 276 days. I do not need to turn on the lights to locate the bed. How long I sleep, I'm not sure, but when I wake, it is with a start. My thoughts are focused on the Pacific Islander in *Moby-Dick*. Having cast the fortune-telling bones on deck, he sees in them his death. Folding his arms, he awaits its coming.

When I get to the ward, light from the adjacent building silhouettes his frame. Every now and then, a tremor moves the silhouette. Convinced that in the hours to come he has a rendezvous to keep, a rock sits alone, waiting.

## That's It

Since the Stephanio Fassio episode, my interactions with my medical division's chief of service have been both few and brief.

One involved the hospital administrator's concerns about my frequent trips to his office complaining about the lack of nursing care on the ward.

That meeting terminated with the chief saying, "The hospital administrator would appreciate seeing you a little less frequently. However, I suggested a way that the desired outcome could be achieved."

Translated, that meant that for the rest of my internship, whatever ward I was on would be guaranteed RN coverage, instead of one nurse covering two or even sometimes three wards.

The only other time that I had been summoned to his office was following an incident in which I berated an attending for his lack of medical knowledge. Again, the conversation was precise and to the point. "I want you to be more diplomatic when you challenge an attending. Think very, very seriously about a written apology: not because you were wrong, but, because you were disrespectful."

I anticipated the first two summonses to his office. But this one … If shit is going to fly, I have no idea why.

Two other individuals are seated in the room. I recognize one as the chief from Fourth Division.

Introductions are made, in which I learn that the third person is the assistant medical director for the Fourth Medical Division.

When asked if I remember Samuel Cheney, all I can think of is, *Why Samuel Cheney?*

"Yes," I reply. "Samuel Cheney, an eighty-one- or eighty-two-year-old dumped onto our service at midnight by the Fourth Division admitting officer, had metastatic cancer to his left pleura"

The word *dumped* causes a predictable effect. Facial muscles tighten ever so slightly.

"Do you remember his diagnosis?"

I answer: "Yes: Adenocarcinoma of the tail of the pancreas, metastatic to the left pleura."

At this point, the Fourth Division attending suddenly interrupts. "How did you know precisely where the primary tumor was and what the diagnosis was? You only had him for eight hours."

There is now no mistaking it. I have an "I want to hear this one" audience.

I script the answer with my boss in mind.

"On X-ray, Mr. Cheney came in with a total white-out of only his left lung. There was absolutely no fluid on the right. The fluid removed from his chest was bloody. After treatment with potassium hydroxide, microscopic examination revealed clumps of epithelial cells consistent with an adenocarcinoma. Had the cancer spread through the bloodstream, both lungs would have been involved. The only way you can get unilateral left pleural involvement is by lymphatic drainage. The only retroperitoneal epithelial organ that has the appropriate lymphatic drainage is the pancreas, more specifically, the tail of the pancreas."

The two visitors get up, thank my boss, and leave.

I look at my chief of service. "That's it?"

"That's it."

Pushing two sheets of paper across the desk, he adds, "This is a contract for a first-year residency position on the First Medical Division, should you decide to stay."

The paper has not yet reached the end of his desk when I reply. "May I please have a pen?"

## The Ugliest Man in the World

What should have been recognizable as the head of a human being is but a skull, over which is drawn a taut conglomerate patchwork of thin, glossy, hairless, grafted skin and scar tissue. Having neither ears nor hair to speak of, and only a vestige of a nose, his face is a grotesque abstract. Whoever has had to fashion a face had little to work with.

With two seriously ill patients already admitted to the ward, it's necessary to determine how critical immediate medical intervention is for this patient. Henry Roberts has been sent in because of progressive loss of appetite, weakness, and an enlarged liver. As I quickly examine the patient, I make an initial working diagnosis. My hand probing his abdomen tells me of a large, non-tender liver, studded with numerous hard nodules. I know that he will keep until my other patients are out of the woods. Unless I can document an alternative diagnosis, there will be little that I can do for him.

The need to communicate to a patient through the sound of one's voice and what can only be termed *the laying on of hands*, the unspoken words that say, "I understand your anguish and your fright" never happened. When I walk away from this patient, I do not even try. I have already seen a lot of things but never before a human so mutilated as to be alien.

It's already dusk when I push Henry Roberts's bed from the ward into the examination room. I do not turn the lights on. We both exist there in the semi-darkness, quietly talking, he propped up in the bed, myself half-sitting, half-standing on its edge. At first, the conversation consists only of replies to my questions and verbal reassurances. For a patient to answer honestly, he must face those fathomless fears that come from knowing that something is wrong and that he is powerless to right it.

Communication is not a problem. Henry Roberts has already made his own diagnosis and now only hopes that he is wrong. If left this thin gossamer of hope, he may be better able to endure his last days. As he opens up, I merely have to guide him from one area to another as he relates first the history of his disease and then of his life.

In the semi-darkness, I hear a saga that has its beginnings in the battles of the Atlantic and the North Sea—of a time when men and ships tried to overwhelm the destructive power of the enemy with numbers; of ships at the periphery of a convoy suddenly becoming explosive beacons in the night; of nights of fearing the darkness …

Once, his ship picked up survivors from a U-boat. When asked how he felt toward those men, Henry Roberts is a little taken aback. "They were like us. They had a job to do."

Three times his ship goes down. It is the last time when his ordeal begins. The convoy was made up of a core of fifteen merchant ships and two destroyer escorts. With luck, some would have gotten through.

Luck is something this convoy was not to have. The U-boats had rendezvoused and were waiting. When the Royal Navy arrived, all that remains were two half-dead survivors.

Who they were was not important; what they stood for was. If humanly possible, they were to be saved.

For Henry Roberts, a face had to be made. He had been on aboard a tanker. Although he survived the initial explosion, fire had consumed his face. Nine years and forty-five operations later, a functional face was constructed for him. His face is to be a collective tribute to those who worked on him, yet it bears little resemblance to anything human.

Rounds at his bedside become shorter and shorter. Those who come to visit him are mirrors of the things my eyes alone cannot see. Their depth and warmth confer to him a status not commonly found. He cares deeply for the world beyond his personal domain. He is a giver without the telltale hesitation.

It's ironic. The young children and even the adolescents who visit him are obviously very fond of him; yet Mr. Roberts told me that, in the past, they were often his cruelest tormentors. While others pretend not to see or turn away, to the children of the neighborhood his appearance was often a source of sport. Half in jest, half in earnest, he once turned to the bulldog that shared his cast in life and said, "You're the ugliest dog in the world and I'm the ugliest man in the world. We deserve each other."

As his condition deteriorates, his bed progressively moves from seventh on the right to "launching pad."

Thursday morning, he makes a request to see his dog. The attending physician's face searches mine to see if I am ready to accept the possibility that granting this request may precipitate Henry Roberts's death. Each day has documented the certainty of his demise, yet the infinitesimal possibility of his having a remedial disease holds sway for a moment and then is extinguished.

Four of his friends are waiting. With them is a big, mostly white English bulldog. At first, the dog pays little attention to the figure fifty yards away. Then something about the figure in the wheelchair catches his attention. His huge head bends forward, as if trying to focus better. When sure, he physically drags those trying to hold him.

A rambunctious, exuberant white tail churns in ecstasy. I am surprised at the brevity of the meeting. After a few minutes, Mr. Roberts reaches out, takes my hand, and draws me down to him. "We had better go."

He turns for a last time at the door to see his dog frantically pull against the efforts of two grown men struggling to hold him.

As I am leaving the ward, Mr. Roberts beckons me over. "Are you off duty tonight?"

I answer, "Yes."

"I want to say good-bye." As I turn away in self-defense, "And above all, thank you."

Standing in the hallway of the ward, I try desperately to remember a poem written by an unknown British soldier during World War I.

*Oh God, when death is near*
*let me mock the haggard face of fear*
*that when I fall if fall I must,*

*my soul may triumph in the dust.*

An hour later the telephone rings. On the six o'clock nurse's rounds, Henry Eldridge Roberts was found without pulse, blood pressure, respiration …

A Native American prayer that my father taught me finds a voice.

*Make me always ready to come to you*
*with clean hands and straight eyes,*
*so when life fades as a fading sunset*
*my spirit may come to you without shame.*

## Sunday Morning

Sunday morning is one of those days when a quiet moment is welcome. Henry Roberts still roams in and out of my thoughts. It takes a very special person to live with his alienation yet have his humanity flourish.

It's starting to rain. The rain takes the form of circles. They tenaciously cling to glass as we do to life. In the past, men of philosophy, like Pythagoras, Plato, Aristotle, became men of science. Nowadays, men of science occasionally become philosophers. Medicine, more than any other area of science, takes one back full circle.

The dawn will outlive the drops of rain, and they will be gone, one circle temporarily replacing another. The morning sun does not forget to arrive. The sun measures the day. The moon measures the seasons. Is death but part of the seeming timelessness of existence?

It will soon be a year. In that time, I have learned a lot about disease and maybe something about death and dying. You meet many persons who desperately cling to lives that have long lost their substance. Physical existence is the last possession they have. And then, there are those who come to death, "their cups filled."

When you witness it enough, death's finality begins to fade. There is a fleeting glimpse of something beyond death: a circle of birth, death, and again birth that seems to imply eternity. Birth out of death may not be a cliché but rather an observation from those with eyes that see into the cosmology of life that enriches those who have the privilege of a physical tomorrow. The *Kabbalah Law of Tikkun* speaks of life as a cassette that you rewind and play again in a different form with the changes forged in the life just ended.

When this year started, it was all about me. As the year ends, it is more about them. I have learned many facts and concepts about the physical body. In exchange for what healing I could give, my patients have taught me not to treat them as a diseased lung or kidney but to understand that disease occurs in unique individuals. I need to go beyond the physical body if I want to be a true healer.

With immense gratitude, my professors of light within the shadows of death are sincerely thanked.

## The Poem

In Bellevue's medical library, a poem written in 1918 by a nurse, Mary St John hangs in a relatively obscure corner. When I first read it, I considered its verses quaint. Now that I'll be leaving Bellevue to do my military service at the National Institutes of Health, it speaks to me in a different way.

*If your walls could but tell the story*
*Of the deeds of those mighty men,*
*That have traver'st the boards of Bellevue's wards,*
*T'would a wonderful story pen.*

*It would tell of their work and the efforts*
*That were made for the human race;*
*And of each plan that they made to save man,*
*By scribing disease to efface.*

*Then, again it would speak of nurses,*
*Who never once seemed to tire,*
*But would work with their might both day and night,*
*To benefit man, their desire.*

*For this body of earnest, hard workers,*

*With their heart and soul, and brain,*
*Were part of God's plan found in the vain*
*Of the army that's lived not in vain.*

*They would tell how your doors have been open*
*To the sick, the sore, and the sad.*
*How the poor and forsaken you've always taken,*
*And given the best that you've had.*

*How you have never rebuked nor condemned them*
*Because success they did not win.*
*But have unbarred your gates no matter how late,*
*And always have welcomed them in.*

*That these walls so shall be silence,*
*Whose stories must then pass away,*
*Means a sorrow, this coming to-morrow,*
*For the ones who know them today.*

*And when in dust you have been leveled,*
*Your requiem song has been sung;*
*In memory's hall will be found on the wall,*
*A tablet to Bellevue there hung.*